AF307207

R. J. Gralla   M. Tonato   F. Roila   (Eds.)

Perugia Consensus Conference on Antiemetic Therapy

Springer

*Berlin
Heidelberg
New York
Barcelona
Budapest
Hong Kong
London
Milan
Paris
Singapore
Tokyo*

R. J. Gralla   M. Tonato   F. Roila   (Eds.)

Perugia Consensus Conference on Antiemetic Therapy

With 5 Illustrations and 19 Tables

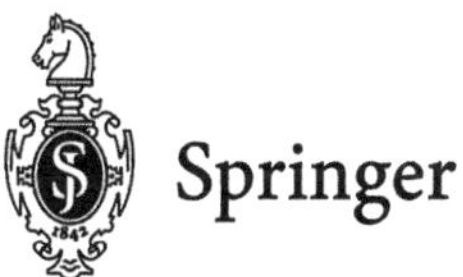 Springer

Richard J. Gralla
Ochsner Cancer Institute
1514 Jefferson Highway
New Orleans, LA 70121-2483, U.S.A

Tel.:   +1-504-842-3261
Fax: +1-504-842-4533

Maurizio Tonato
Oncologia Medica, Policlinico Monteluce
Via Brunamonti
06122 Perugia, Italy

Tel.:   +39-75-5783456
Fax: +39-75-5720990
e-mail: oncmedpg@krenet.it

Fausto Roila
Oncologia Medica, Policlinico Monteluce
Via Brunamonti
06122 Perugia, Italy

Tel.:   +39-75-5783456
Fax: +39-75-5720990
e-mail: oncmedpg@krenet.it

ISBN-13: 978-3-642-72139-7   e-ISBN-13: 978-3-642-72137-3
DOI: 10.1007/978-3-642-72137-3

Library of Congress Cataloging-in-Publication Data
Perugia Consensus Conference on Antiemetic Therapy (1997)
  Perugia Consensus Conference on Antiemetic Therapy / R.J. Gralla, M. Tonato, F. Roila, (eds.).
  "This conference ... was also the fifth conference in a successful series, the Perugia International
Cancer Conference (PICC V)"--Pref. Includes bibliographical references and index.
  ISBN-13: 978-3-642-72139-7
  1. Cancer--Chemotherapy--Complications--Chemotherapy--Congresses. 2. Antineoplastic agents--
Side-effects--Chemotherapy--Congresses. 3. Antiemetics--Congresses. 4. Nausea--Chemotherapy--
Congresses. 5. Vomiting--Chemotherapy--Congresses. I. Gralla, Richard J. II. Tonato, M. (Maurizio)
III. Roila, F. (Fausto), 1953-   . IV. Perugia International Cancer Conference (5th : 1997) V. Title.
[DNLM: 1. Antiemetics--therapeutic use congresses. 2. Neoplasms--drug therapy congresses. 3.
Neoplasms--radiography congresses. QV 73 P471p 1998]   RC271.C5P45   1998   616.99'4061--dc21

Cover design: de'blik, Berlin
Typesetting: I. Gundermann, Springer-Verlag, Heidelberg
SPIN: 10574124   19/3133 – 5 4 3 2 1 0 - Printed on acid-free paper

Preface

In the past decade important progress has been achieved in the prevention of chemotherapy-induced nausea and vomiting, especially after the introduction of 5-HT$_3$ antagonists, which, when used in combination with steroids, can assure significant protection in the majority of patients. Nonetheless, some relevant clinical problems remain without satisfactory answers, and there are major differences in clinical practice regarding antiemetic use.

The reasons for this are numerous, but the lack of reliable data derived from well-conducted clinical trials and difficulties in transferring the results of clinical research to daily practice are probably the most important. Furthermore, some methodological aspects of the research in this area are still not well defined, and this accounts for the lack of clear evidence in favour of a definitive choice in controversial issues.

Consensus methods provide a useful way of identifying and measuring uncertainty in medical research and can be used as aids to decision-making in clinical practice. Considering all these facts, the Subcommittee for Antiemetics of the Multinational Association of Supportive Care in Cancer (MASCC) decided, during the Congress held in Luxembourg in September 1995, to organize a consensus conference on the use of antiemetics.

To identify the most important topics on which a consensus should be measured and developed, the subcommittee elaborated and circulated a questionnaire among experts. The results of this survey have recently been published [1], and eight major issues were identified that would constitute the basis for the conference. This conference was held in Perugia, Italy on 28-29 April 1997, under the auspices of MASCC, of the European Society of Medical Oncology (ESMO), and of the Italian Association of Medical Oncology (AIOM). It was also the fifth conference in a successful series, the Perugia International Cancer Conference (PICC V).

The meeting was organized in eight sessions, corresponding exactly to the topics outlined in the questionnaire:
1. The 5-HT$_3$ receptor antagonists in the prevention of acute emesis induced by cisplatin and moderately emetogenic chemotherapy: problems of dose, schedule, and route

2. Other antiemetic agents: corticosteroids, dopamine antagonists and others
3. Delayed emesis, emesis induced by multiple-day chemotherapy, and rescue antiemetic treatment
4. Special problems: emesis in children undergoing chemotherapy and emesis due to radiation therapy
5. Other emetic problems: anticipatory emesis, emesis induced by high-dose chemotherapy and by opiates
6. Methodology of trials: response categories, emetogenic classifications of antineoplastic agents, and methodology to study a new antiemetic agent
7. Statistical considerations: power of study and number of patients to be enrolled, prognostic factors, multiple cycles of chemotherapy, and delayed emesis
8. Neuropharmacology: serotonin antagonists and the current understanding of the pathophysiology of emesis

Furthermore, the subcommittee decided that, for each session, a discussant would provide a written review of a topic that had been submitted to a respondent and to the chairman of the session. This document, together with the respondent's comments, was given to all the meeting participants to prepare for the discussion.

At the end of the discussion, the panel of each session prepared the consensus document. Common criteria were used to prepare the final documents; in particular, each topic requiring a consensus was evaluated according to the scientific confidence level and to the consensus level among the panel.

The level of scientific confidence was classified as High: repeated, randomized trials that were appropriately sized and well conducted; Moderate: at least one randomized trial supported by well-conducted phase II trials, or possibly several well-conducted phase II studies; Low: formal clinical trials of a level less than that expressed above; Very low: clinical impression only; and No confidence possible. The well-defined topics, the world-renowned experts, the stimulating atmosphere, and the open discussion made the Perugia Consensus Conference a very productive one.

The papers of the single sessions were prepared in a relatively short time, thanks to the spirit of collaboration of all participants, and this makes this publication a document which we hope will be worthy of consideration and useful as a basis for future developments.

Richard J. Gralla
Maurizio Tonato
Fausto Roila

Reference
1. Ballatori E, Roila F, De Angelis V et al (1997) Clinical and methodological issues in antiemetic therapy: a worldwide survey of experts' opinions. Support Care Cancer 5 : 269-273

Contents

List of Contributors

M. S. Aapro, M. D.
Institut Multidisciplinaire d'Oncologie
Clinique de Grenolier
CH-1272 Grenolier

P. L. R. Andrews, Ph. D.
Department of Physiology
St. George's Hospital Medical School, Tooting
London, SW17 0RE, UK

E. Ballatori, M. D.
University of L'Aquila
Department of Internal Medicine and Public Health
Medical Statistics Unit
I-L'Aquila

P. H. M. De Mulder, M. D.
University Hospital Nijmegen
Division of Medical Oncology 550
Geert Groteplein 8, NL-6510 HB Nijmegen

A. Del Favero, M. D.
Instituto Di Medicina Interna E. Scienze Oncologiche
Policlinico Monteluce
Via Brunamonti, I-06122 Perugia

M. A. Dicato, M. D.
Hematology-Oncology
Centre Hospitalier
L-1210 Luxembourg

A. du Bois, M. D.
St. Vincentius Hospital
D-76137 Karlsruhe

M. J. Edelman, M. D.
VA Northern California Health Care System
150 Muir Road # 1511
Martinez, CA 94553-4612, USA

P. C. Feyer, M. D., Ph. D.
Department of Radiotherapy
Medical School Charité
Humboldt University Berlin
Schumannstraße 20/21, D-10117 Berlin

D. R. Gandara, M. D.
U. C. Davis Cancer Center
4501 X Street
Sacramento, CA 95817, USA

R. J. Gralla, M. D.
Ochsner Cancer Institute
1514 Jefferson Highway
New Orleans, LA 70121-2483, USA

S. Groshen, Ph. D.
Universtiy of South California School of Medicine
Norris Comprehensive Cancer Center
Department of Preventive Medicine
Los Angeles, CA, USA

S. M. Grunberg, M. D.
Department of Medicine and Pharmacology
University of Vermont
Burlington, VT, USA

J. Herrstedt, M. D.
Department of Oncology R
Copenhagen University Hospital Herlev
Herlev Ringvej
DK-2730 Herlev

P. J. Hesketh, M. D.
Section of Medical Oncology
St. Elizabeth's Medical Center
736 Cambrigde Street
Boston, MA 02135, USA

H. E. Hynes, M. D.
Wichita CCOP
Wichita, KA, USA

R. A. Joss (†)
Department of Medicine
Kantonsspital
CH-6000 Lucerne 16

J. J. Kirshner, M. D.
Syracuse Hematology-Oncology CCOP
Syracuse, NY, USA

M. G. Kris, M. D.
Thoracic Oncology Service
Division of Solid Tumor Oncology
Department of Medicine
Memorial Sloan-Kettering Cancer Center and
Cornell University Medical College
New York, NY, USA

M. Marty, M. D.
Department of Medical Oncology
Hospital Saint-Louis
1, avenue Claude Vellefaux
F-75475 Paris Cedex 10

G. R. Morrow, Ph. D., M. S.
University of Rochester Cancer Center
Rochester, NY, USA

R. J. Naylor, M. D.
Postgraduate Studies in Pharmacology
The School of Pharmacy
University of Bradford
Bradford, West Yorkshire, BD7 1DP, UK

I. Olver, M. D.
Royal Adelaide Hospital Cancer Centre
Adelaide, South Australia
Australia

E. A. Perez, M. D.
Mayo Clinic
Jacksonville
4500 San Pablo Road
Jacksonville, FL 32224-1865, USA

F. Roila, M. D.
Oncologia Medica
Policlinico Monteluce
Via Brunamonti, I-06122 Perugia

J. A. Roscoe
University of Rochester Cancer Center
601 Elmwood Ave. # 704
Rochester, NY 14642-0001, USA

R. J. Rosenbluth, M. D.
Northern New Jersey CCOP
Hackensack, NJ, USA

J. F. Smyth, M. D.
Department of Clinical Oncology
Western General Hospital
University of Edinburgh
Edinburgh, Scotland

T. R. Spitzer, M. D.
Bone Marrow Transplant Program
Department of Medicine
Massachussetts General Hospital
Boston, MA 02114, USA

A. L. Stewart, M. D.
Department of Clinical Oncology (Radiotherapy)
Christie Hospital and Holt Radium Institute
Wilmslow Road, Manchester M20 9BX, UK

O. J. Titlbach, M. D., Ph. D.
  Department of Medicine I
  Hospital Friedrichshain
  Landsberger Allee 49, D-10249 Berlin

M. Tonato, M. D.
  Oncologia Medica
  Policlinico Monteluce
  Via Brunamonti, I-06122 Perugia

D. Warr, M. D.
  Ontario Cancer Institute
  Princess Margaret Hospital
  610 University Avenue
  Toronto, Ontario M5G 2M9, Canada

Corticosteroids, Dopamine Antagonists, and Other Drugs

Jørn Herrstedt, Matti S. Aapro, John F. Smyth, Albano Del Favero

ABSTRACT The literature on corticosteroids, dopamine antagonists, and other antiemetics, such as cannabinoids and benzodiazepines, was reviewed and presented at a consensus conference on antiemetics. Based on the reviews and the discussion during the conference, guidelines for the use of these agents are given.

Introduction

The selective serotonin (5-HT_3) receptor antagonists have dramatically improved the treatment of acute chemotherapy-induced nausea and vomiting. This has, to some extent, diverted attention from other potentially useful antiemetics (Table 1). The complete control rate of cancer chemotherapy-induced nausea and vomiting is still insufficient, however, as patients sustain acute (20–40% incidence) [103] and delayed emesis (22–89% incidence) [2] as well as lack of total control after several cycles of chemotherapy [29]. We need even more effective agents and combinations of agents if we are to obtain maximum quality of life for our patients. It is important to appreciate that total and not partial control of emesis is considered by most patients to be the only clearly significant benefit from antiemetic treatment [10].

Corticosteroids

Historical Background

Chemotherapy cycles containing prednisone in the original alternating cycles of MOPP/MOP [115] were better tolerated than those not containing steroids. This and other serendipitous observations led to pilot studies using corticosteroids to protect against chemotherapy-induced emesis (reviewed in [1]). Animal studies confirming these clinical data have been performed, and prevention of cisplatin-induced emesis by corticosteroids has been observed in ferrets and dogs [27, 81].

Table 1 Classification of antiemetics

Serotonin antagonists	Ondansetron Granisetron Tropisetron Dolasetron
Corticosteroids	Dexamethasone Methylprednisolone
Dopamine antagonists Phenothiazines	Prochlorperazine Chlorpromazine Metopimazine
Butyrophenones	Haloperidol Droperidol
Butyrophenone derivative	Domperidone
Substituted benzamides	Metoclopramide Alizapride Clebopride
Cannabinoids	Nabilone Dronabinol Levonantradol
Benzodiazepines	Lorazepam Diazepam
Antihistamines	Diphenhydramine
Anticholinergics	Scopolamine
Miscellaneous	Tricyclic antidepressants Histamine H_2 antagonists ACTH

Comparative Studies of Corticosteroids Alone Against Other Agents or Placebo in Acute Emesis

Twelve out of 26 studies published until 1990 [1] indicated that corticosteroids were superior to the comparative agent, and many "negative studies" showed that corticosteroids often had a similar effect to an efficacious but less well-tolerated antiemetic. In double-blind crossover studies, patients indicated a preference for the treatment course containing corticosteroids. These positive studies were limited to patients treated with chemotherapy containing no or low-dose (less than 50 mg/m^2) cisplatin and led many groups to believe that corticosteroids should be used alone for first-line antiemetic prophylaxis of moderately emetogenic chemotherapy. Such a position was further reinforced by the observation that when "appropriate" high doses of corticosteroids (namely 8 mg dexamethasone i.v. before chemotherapy, followed by 4 mg p.o. four times a day on days 1 and 2 and tapering off on days 3–5) were compared with ondansetron (4 mg i.v. followed by 4 mg orally every 6 h on days 1–5), patients treated with dexamethasone and undergoing moderately emetogenic chemotherapy experienced the same rate of acute antiemetic protection with either agent and a better protection against delayed nausea and vomiting while taking dexamethasone [62]. A major study encompassing 428 patients has now shown that dexamethasone (8 mg i.v. before moderately emetogenic chemotherapy, plus 4 mg orally for four doses every 6 h) alone provides a 49% complete protection rate against nausea and vomiting, while 3 mg granisetron i.v. gives a 43% complete protection rate and the combination of both agents provides a 70% complete protection rate [61].

Corticosteroids Added to Other Antiemetic Agents for Control of Acute Emesis

Controlled studies described in 22 reports were reviewed in 1990 [1]. Seventeen reports indicate a minor or major benefit in antiemetic control thanks to the addition of steroids to other non-5-HT$_3$ receptor antagonists.

Those studies that were considered insufficiently positive ("not reaching statistical significance") were often small studies, where a difference is easy to miss. It was concluded that corticosteroid-based antiemetic combinations provide significantly better control of chemotherapy-induced nausea and vomiting than non-steroid-based combinations, and in the late 1980s the standard treatment given to control acute nausea and vomiting was a combination of metoclopramide, corticosteroids and agents to counteract the side effects of metoclopramide. All presently available 5-HT$_3$ receptor antagonists (dolasetron, granisetron, ondansetron, and tropisetron) have been tested in randomized studies alone or in combination with corticosteroids, mainly for the control of cisplatin-induced emesis, but also for control of moderately emetogenic chemotherapy-induced nausea and vomiting. All these studies have shown that corticosteroids increase the rate of antiemetic control over that obtained with a 5-HT$_3$ receptor antagonist alone [112]. A study in the ferret has shown that while the number of animals that experience no emesis is not increased by the use of dexamethasone, the total number of emetic episodes is reduced [104].

Corticosteroids Alone or Combined with Other Agents for Control of Delayed Emesis

As reviewed elsewhere [2], ACTH has been shown to decrease the delayed emesis experienced by patients undergoing cisplatin-containing chemotherapy compared with placebo. Dexamethasone has also been shown to be superior to placebo in such settings, and the combination of dexamethasone and metoclopramide has been recommended as a possible standard for the prevention of delayed nausea and vomiting. Many studies have recently compared the role of dexamethasone alone or dexamethasone combined with 5-HT$_3$ receptor antagonists for control of delayed emesis related to both highly and moderately emetogenic chemotherapy, and this issue is discussed elsewhere in this volume.

Limitations to the Use of Corticosteroids as Antiemetics

Corticosteroids can decompensate diabetes or induce psychosis even when given in a single administration. They might reactivate a duodenal or gastric ulcer [12], but this is unlikely in very short-term use. The side effects related to long-term use of corticosteroids are not limiting factors in the antiemetic setting. One group has shown no significant hypothalamic-pituitary-adrenal suppression in cancer patients after a 4-week treatment with methylprednisolone [74].

Concern has been raised about the immunosuppressive effects of corticosteroids [47, 48]. While it is commonly felt that most antitumor chemotherapies are already highly immunosuppressive by themselves, and cancer patients do exhibit variable degrees of immunosuppression, dexamethasone has been shown to suppress natural cytotoxic cell activity [99]. The antitumor activity of cisplatin, either in a mouse model or in vitro, is not decreased by dexamethasone [4]. In line with previously expressed concern about possible harmful effects of corticosteroids in some cancer patients are one historical observation [107] and a more recent one, which show a modification of the metastatic pattern in breast cancer patients who receive long-term low-dose steroids [77].

Side Effects of Corticosteroids as Antiemetics

Insomnia, euphoria, or anxiety might actually occur with the same frequency as with prochlorperazine, an agent that induces significantly more somnolence [17]. Facial flush is often reported with methylprednisolone, and several papers report pharyngeal or perineal itch (reviewed in [1]) when dexamethasone is infused rapidly. A single report of a case of acute posterior subcapsular cataracts has been published. ACTH may cause melanodermia in a few patients. In children, the use of corticosteroids is quite frequent in the therapy of CNS tumors, and the long-term side effects of such prolonged usage are well known. It is therefore not surprising that some pediatric oncologists have voiced concern about their use.

Mechanism of Action

The antiemetic action of corticosteroids is not yet understood, but several hypotheses have been suggested. The recently developed animal studies mentioned above might provide a useful model to explore this. No increase of plasma prostaglandins has been observed in patients undergoing cisplatin treatment [108], and thus an antiprostaglandin effect is improbable. Corticosteroids might modify the capillary permeability of the chemoreceptor trigger zone [75], stabilize some membrane or intracellular components (lysosomes), or decrease some of the inflammatory changes in the gut after chemotherapy. It has also been suggested that they may play a role in endorphin release [50]. Recent evidence points to the possibility of increased activity of steroids in patients who have low endogenous cortisol excretion [32, 35, 59].

Dose Schedule of Corticosteroids as Antiemetics

There is no agreement on the best dose schedule of corticosteroids used for antiemesis. Single-agent dexamethasone is active at a dose of 8 mg i.v., with no improvement of results when doses are raised to 32 mg [30]. There is no difference in activity between 40 mg methylprednisolone i.v. and 125 mg t.i.d. [20]. We speculate that steroids should be started several hours before chemotherapy [67] and we frequently taper off doses over 2 days rather than stopping abruptly, as some patients complain of myalgias or recurrent vomiting after abrupt discontinuation of steroids [3].

Guidelines (Table 2)

Acute Emesis, Moderately or Highly Emetogenic Chemotherapy
As (a) many studies have shown that 5-HT$_3$ receptor antagonists alone are as efficacious as, if not superior to non-5-HT$_3$-containing antiemetic combinations, (b) dexamethasone in some studies is superior to 5-HT$_3$ receptor antagonists in the control of moderately emetogenic chemotherapy, and (c) all studies show that corticosteroids enhance the antiemetic activity of other agents, it can be stated that patients treated with moderately and highly emetogenic chemotherapy should receive a combination of steroids and 5-HT$_3$ receptor antagonists for acute-phase antiemetic prophylaxis.

Delayed Emesis
Corticosteroids alone or in combination with other agents should be used for control of delayed emesis.

However, because of some concern about a negative effect of corticosteroids on the long-term relapse pattern of breast cancer, their indiscriminate

Table 2 Level of confidence and consensus concerning corticosteroids

Level of consensus	Moderately emetogenic chemotherapy	Level of confidence
High	Equal or superior to non-5-HT$_3$ antagonists in prevention of acute emesis. Less toxicity	High
Moderate	Equal to 5-HT$_3$ antagonists in prevention of acute emesis	Moderate
High	Enhance the effect of other antiemetics in prevention of acute emesis	High
Moderate	Effective when used alone or in combination with another agent in prevention of delayed emesis	Low

Level of consensus	Highly emetogenic chemotherapy	Level of confidence
High	Enhance the effect of 5-HT$_3$ antagonists including high-dose metoclopramide in prevention of acute emesis	High
High	Effective when used alone or in combination with another agent in prevention of delayed emesis	Moderate

Level of consensus	General comments	Level of confidence
High	Optimal dose/schedule unknown	High
High	No difference in effect or toxicity between corticosteroids	Low
High	Toxicity seldom prohibits use	Moderate

use during the curative treatment of nonhematological malignancies may be open to some question.

Dopamine Antagonists

Dopamine D$_2$ receptor antagonists, especially the phenothiazines, were the mainstay of antiemetic therapy from the 1950s to the early 1980s. The dopamine antagonists could be classified as phenothiazines, butyrophenones (plus the derivative domperidone), or substituted benzamides (Table 1).

Substituted Benzamides

Metoclopramide is one of the most thoroughly investigated antiemetics; the efficacy of high doses in patients receiving cisplatin-based chemotherapy is well documented [41, 52, 58, 106]. It is now recognized that the antiemetic effect of high doses of metoclopramide is probably due to 5-HT$_3$ receptor antagonism [85], whereas adverse events, and the effect of low doses, are due to antagonism of the dopamine D$_2$ receptor. In doses of 2 mg/kg $\times$ 5 [41] or 3 mg/kg $\times$ 2 [69] i.v., metoclopramide prevents emesis in 30–40% of patients receiving cisplatin-based chemotherapy. High-dose metoclopramide is superior to steroids in patients receiving 50 mg/m^2 or more of cisplatin [1], but clearly inferior to the 5-HT$_3$ receptor antagonists [19, 80]. Results in patients receiving moderately emetogenic chemotherapy are difficult to interpret; there seems to be no advantage of high versus "conventional" doses of metoclopramide. The effect of high, antiserotonergic doses of metoclopramide will not be further addressed. Early studies of metoclopramide were uncontrolled [65] or compared metoclopramide with placebo [23, 86, 90, 97, 114], prochlorperazine [7, 9, 37], metopimazine [86], domperidone [8, 25, 31, 38, 68, 101, 109, 117], a steroid [8, 25, 97, 101, 102], or a cannabinoid [22, 33]. Recent studies have compared metoclopramide with ondansetron [13, 64, 79] and dolasetron [34].

An uncontrolled study [65] yielded the observation that a single oral dose of 20 mg metoclopramide was effective in 92% of patients receiving cisplatin-based chemotherapy. This is in glaring contrast to other studies, in which metoclopramide in doses of 20 mg $\times$ 3 or 4 p.o. was ineffective and not superior to placebo [114] or prochlorperazine [7, 9]. In a double-blind study [37] conducted in 100 patients, 3 $\times$ 20 mg metoclopramide was slightly superior to 3 $\times$ 10 mg prochlorperazine, but both were largely ineffective as 74% and 92% of the patients vomited. Studies comparing high and low doses of metoclopramide show that low i.v. doses of metoclopramide are ineffective in cisplatin-based chemotherapy [52, 94], as only 7–10% are protected from emesis.

In patients receiving moderately emetogenic chemotherapy, the use of low oral doses of metoclopramide is just as questionable. Metoclopramide (10–20 mg $\times$ 3) was not significantly different from placebo [86, 90] and was inferior to domperidone [25], dexamethasone [25], and dronabinol [33]. In one study, the oral dose of metoclopramide was increased to 0.5 mg/kg $\times$ 4, and the antiemetic effect then became similar to that of domperidone [68]. Metoclopramide (20 mg $\times$ 5 i.v.) was reported to be equivalent to methylprednisolone (125 mg $\times$ 3) in three studies [8, 101, 102]. In two of these studies, a comparison with domperidone was included, and metoclopramide was superior in patients receiving CMF [101] but not in those receiving doxorubicin [8]. Single intravenous doses of 10–20 mg metoclopramide were not different from

placebo in effect [97] or were equal [31, 117] or inferior [38, 109] to single doses of domperidone, and inferior to multiple doses of dexamethasone [97]. In
three recent trials, metoclopramide given as a loading dose of 60–80 mg i.v.
followed by 20 mg × 3 p.o. was compared with the 5-HT$_3$ receptor antagonist
ondansetron [13, 64, 79]. Ondansetron was superior in two studies [13, 64],
whereas no significant differences between the agents was seen in the third
study [79]. Based on the studies above, it is possible that an increase in the
oral maintenance dose of metoclopramide could have improved the antiemetic efficacy of the metoclopramide regimen.

In conclusion, low oral and i.v. doses of metoclopramide are ineffective in
patients receiving cisplatin-based chemotherapy. In moderately emetogenic
chemotherapy, repeated i.v. doses of 20 mg possess antiemetic activity, whereas the effect of oral doses of 20 mg is questionable. There is no discrepancy
in this observation, because the oral bioavailability of metoclopramide ranges from 30% to 100% with a median of 60–80% [15].

Other substituted benzamides include alizapride and clebopride. At present they seem to have no advantage over metoclopramide [11, 63, 98, 116].

Phenothiazines

Chlorpromazine was the the first phenothiazine that had a demonstrated antiemetic effect. When administered i.m. in doses of 25 mg × 4, chlorpromazine is comparable to high-dose metoclopramide in patients receiving moderately emetogenic chemotherapy, but inferior to it against cisplatin-induced
emesis [24]. The phenothiazines include thiethylperazine, thiopropazate,
perphenazine, metopimazine, and prochlorperazine, with the latter being the
most frequently investigated and most commonly used of the agents.

Prochlorperazine in oral doses of 5–10 mg × 2–4 is superior to placebo [36,
88] in patients receiving 5-FU, equal to metopimazine [87], equal [36] or inferior [95, 105] to delta-9-tetrahydrocannabinol (THC), inferior to nabilone
[5], and equal [39] or inferior [78] to dexamethasone in patients receiving various kinds of moderately emetogenic chemotherapy. In this setting, a single
dose of 10 mg i.v. prochlorperazine plus 10 mg dexamethasone was also inferior to granisetron [113]. In patients receiving low-dose cisplatin-based chemotherapy, prochlorperazine is inferior to nabilone [51], and in patients submitted to high-dose cisplatin prochlorperazine is inferior to high-dose metoclopramide [41].

The antiemetic effect of the piperidine derivative metopimazine has only
been investigated in a few trials. Metopimazine is superior to placebo in oral
doses of 10–15 mg × 3 [60, 87] and equal to prochlorperazine [87], but with significantly less sedation. Metopimazine is safe in oral doses of 30 mg × 4–6 [55],
but the agent has not been investigated in a traditional dose-response study.

Prochlorperazine and metopimazine both have higher affinity for dopamine D_2 receptors than metoclopramide, and in contrast to this agent the effect of high doses is not mediated by antagonist activity at 5-HT$_3$ receptors [49, 53]. None of the phenothiazines is selective for the dopamine D_2 receptor, however. Metopimazine, like chlorpromazine, has a high affinity for α_1-adrenergic receptors, meaning that orthostatic hypotension is the dose-limiting adverse event. Metopimazine, on the other hand, is almost devoid of the extrapyramidal adverse events that are frequently observed with prochlorperazine. Both agents have been investigated in higher doses than originally recommended. Two small studies, one in patients receiving dacarbazine [21] and one in cisplatin-treated patients [111], indicated that the antiemetic potential of metopimazine does increase with dose. Extrapyramidal adverse events were not reported even with very high doses which, in one of the studies [111], caused orthostatic hypotension. Prochlorperazine was investigated in two dose–response studies [16, 92], and the recommended i.v. 0.8 mg/kg $\times$ 2 dose was subsequently compared with 2 mg/kg $\times$ 5 i.v. metoclopramide in 200 patients submitted to cisplatin- or non-cisplatin-based chemotherapy [93]. No significant differences in antiemetic effect were found, but restlessness and moderate to severe sedation were observed in a high proportion of the patients in both regimens.

To conclude, low doses of phenothiazines are not effective in patients receiving cisplatin. There are no data supporting the use of phenothiazines given as single agents, except in patients receiving mildly emetogenic chemotherapy, e.g. 5-FU. Higher doses seem to increase the antiemetic effect, but probably also increase the adverse events, certainly with prochlorperazine.

Butyrophenones

The butyrophenones are not widely used, but haloperidol, droperidol, and domperidone all have antiemetic effects. Domperidone is said not to cross the blood–brain barrier and therefore to be devoid of extrapyramidal adverse events. The drug is not available for i.v. use, owing to the risk of cardiac dysrhythmias. In mild to moderately emetogenic chemotherapy, it is superior to placebo and equal [68] or superior [25] to low doses of metoclopramide. Pilot studies indicated an antiemetic effect of i.m. and i.v. doses of droperidol in patients receiving cisplatin [18, 43, 66]. In a small (patient-blinded) study, droperidol was superior to prochlorperazine in gynecological patients receiving cisplatin. In a double-blind study [52] comparing low-dose metoclopramide plus droperidol plus lorazepam with high-dose metoclopramide plus lorazepam in cisplatin-based chemotherapy, only 10% of the patients in the droperidol plus low-dose metoclopramide arm were protected from vomiting, as against 50% in the high-dose metoclopramide arm. Haloperidol was superior to benzquinamide against emesis induced by cisplatin and nitrogen mustard, but not by doxorubicin [91]. In a randomized, double-blind study, high-dose metoclopramide was only slightly superior to haloperidol given at a dosage of 3 mg × 5 i.v. [45]. To conclude, domperidone has antiemetic activity in patients receiving mildly or moderately emetogenic chemotherapy, whereas droperidol and haloperidol have not been properly investigated in this group of patients. Droperidol and haloperidol both have antiemetic effect in cisplatin-based chemotherapy, but although no direct comparisons have been made, they cannot compete with the 5-HT$_3$ antagonists in terms of efficacy and safety.

Combination of Dopamine Antagonists and Other Antiemetics

Corticosteroids are the antiemetics most frequently used in combination antiemetic therapy. As previously mentioned, steroids significantly improve the antiemetic effect of high-dose metoclopramide [46, 100] and of 5-HT$_3$ receptor antagonists [61, 112]. It is noteworthy that metoclopramide (oral doses of 0.5 mg/kg × 4) plus dexamethasone is more effective than dexamethasone alone in the prevention of delayed emesis resulting from cisplatin-based chemotherapy [71, 89]. Prochlorperazine is especially favorable in combination with dronabinol, because prochlorperazine not only increases the antiemetic effect, but also reduces the dysphoric side effects of cannabinoids [72].

The potential benefit of combining a 5-HT$_3$ antagonist and a dopamine D$_2$ receptor antagonist was emphasized during the Perugia conference in 1990 [44], and recently a few studies have investigated the efficacy of such combinations [14, 28, 54, 56, 57, 73]. Haloperidol was able to improve the antiemetic effect of tropisetron in a trial using historical controls [14]. Three randomized, double-blind studies, one including patients receiving their first course of platinum-based chemotherapy [56] and two including patients refractory to previous antiemetic therapy [28, 54], showed that metopimazine is able to improve the antiemetic effect of ondansetron [54, 56] or of ondansetron plus methylprednisolone [28]. In another double-blind study, metoclopramide improved the efficacy of ondansetron in patients receiving their first course of cisplatin [73]. In an uncontrolled study, the combination of granisetron, dexamethasone, and prochlorperazine prevented acute emesis in as many as 86.7% of patients receiving cisplatin [57]. The effect of a 5-HT$_3$ receptor antagonist plus a corticosteroid plus a dopamine D$_2$ receptor antagonist needs to be investigated in large double-blinded trials.

Other Agents

Cannabinoids

Dronabinol (delta-9-tetrahydrocannabinol) and nabilone are the most frequently investigated cannabinoids. They are active against emesis induced by mild and moderately emetogenic chemotherapy [95, 105] but less effective in patients receiving cisplatin-based chemotherapy [26]. Their use is restricted in some patients, especially the elderly, by adverse events such as somnolence, dysphoria, mental confusion, and hallucinations. A meta-analysis of 750 courses of therapy with dronabinol [96] indicated that the antiemetic effect was maintained, but the frequency of dysphoric adverse events reduced, when the dose was reduced to less than 7 mg/m^2.

We conclude that cannabinoids are effective antiemetics in prevention of acute emesis caused by moderately emetogenic chemotherapy, but they are more toxic than other antiemetics.

Benzodiazepines

The benzodiazepines have primarily been used to reduce adverse events from high-dose metoclopramide [52, 70]. As single agents, the benzodiazepines are not particularly effective, and most trials have focused on the ability to prevent anticipatory nausea and vomiting [42]. A few studies suggest that a benzodiazepine can improve the antiemetic effect of high-dose metoclopramide in patients receiving cisplatin [40], and recently bromazepam improved the effect of ondansetron against emesis induced by carboplatin and cyclophosphamide [82].

Antihistamines and Anticholinergics

Both antihistamines and anticholinergics are primarily effective in the treatment of motion sickness, but also reduce the risk of extrapyramidal adverse events from metoclopramide. In two trials, transdermal scopolamine was no different from placebo [76], but was able to increase the antiemetic effect of metoclopramide plus dexamethasone [84] in patients receiving cisplatin. The combination of granisetron and the antihistamine hydroxyzine hydrochloride resulted in a significantly more pronounced reduction in the intensity of acute nausea than did granisetron alone in head and neck cancer patients undergoing treatment with cisplatin [110].

Table 3 Level of confidence and consensus concerning dopamine antagonists

Level of consensus	Moderately emetogenic chemotherapy	Level of confidence
High	Antiemetic activity in prevention of acute emesis, but less efficacious and more toxic than corticosteroids and 5-HT$_3$ antagonists	Moderate
Moderate	Enhance the effect of 5-HT$_3$ antagonists in prevention of acute emesis	Moderate
Moderate	Enhance the effect of corticosteroids in prevention of delayed emesis	Low
Level of consensus	**Highly emetogenic chemotherapy**	**Level of confidence**
High	Ineffective in prevention of acute emesis when used in low doses	High
High	Antiemetic activity in prevention of acute emesis when used in high doses, but less efficacious and more toxic than 5-HT$_3$ antagonists	Moderate
High	Enhance the effect of 5-HT$_3$ antagonists in prevention of acute emesis	Moderate
High	Enhance the effect of corticosteroids in prevention of delayed emesis	Moderate

Miscellaneous

Antiemetic activity has appeared in small trials with amitriptyline [83] and the histamine H$_2$ antagonist cimetidine [6], but there is no routine indication for the use of these drugs.

Guidelines (Table 3)

Acute Emesis, Highly Emetogenic Chemotherapy

None of the agents reviewed has significant antiemetic activity in patients receiving cisplatin-based chemotherapy when given as single agents in conventional low doses. In high doses, both metoclopramide and prochlorperazine possess an antiemetic effect, but are inferior to the 5-HT$_3$ receptor antagonists in tolerability and efficacy. A 5-HT$_3$ receptor antagonist plus a corticosteroid should therefore be the first choice. Dopamine antagonists have enhanced the antiemetic efficacy of 5-HT$_3$ receptor antagonists in a few trials and have to be evaluated in combination with corticosteroids and 5-HT$_3$ receptor antagonists.

Acute Emesis, Mildly or Moderately Emetogenic Chemotherapy

Single-agent dopamine antagonist therapy is only reasonable in patients receiving mildly emetogenic chemotherapy (e.g., 5-FU). The minimum oral doses of dopamine antagonists, which have shown significant antiemetic effect compared with placebo, are 0.5 mg/kg (or 30 mg) metoclopramide, 5–10 mg prochlorperazine, and 10–15 mg metopimazine, but the dose-finding studies on which this conclusion is based do not comply with recommendations for modern antiemetic trial methodology. In patients receiving moderately emetogenic chemotherapy, a 5-HT$_3$ antagonist plus a corticosteroid should be the first choice. Dopamine antagonist have to be evaluated in combination with corticosteroids and 5-HT$_3$ receptor antagonists.

Delayed Emesis

Few data are available. A corticosteroid should be the first choice. A dopamine antagonist will probably increase the efficacy.

Anticipatory Nausea and Vomiting

Very few data are available. The benzodiazepines might be of use.

Final Comments

This review was presented at a consensus conference on antiemetic therapy in Perugia, 28–29 April 1997. Based on the literature reviewed and the subsequent discussions on the conference, Tables 2 and 3 give recommendations for the use of corticosteroids and dopamine antagonists. The level of confidence and the level of consensus are graded as low, moderate, or high.

References

1. Aapro MS (1991) Present role of corticosteroids as antiemetics. Recent Results Cancer Res 121 : 91–100
2. Aapro MS (1996) Therapeutic approach to delayed emesis. In: Tonato M (ed) Antiemetics in the supportive care of cancer patients. Springer, Berlin Heidelberg New York, pp 73–77
3. Aapro MS, Alberts DS (1981) High-dose dexamethasone for prevention of cisplatin-induced vomiting. Cancer Chemother Pharmacol 7 : 11–14
4. Aapro MS, Alberts DS, Serokman R (1983) Lack of dexamethasone effect on the antitumor activity of cisplatin. Cancer Treat Rep 67 : 1013–1017
5. Ahmedzai S, Carlyle DL, Calder IT, Moran F (1983) Antiemetic efficacy and toxicity of nabilone, a synthetic cannabinoid in lung cancer chemotherapy. Br J Cancer 48 : 657–663

6. Al-Ghamdi MS, Ibrahim EM, Al-Idrissi HY, Al-Khatti AA, Al-Faraj A (1991) Antieme-
    tic efficacy of cimetidine randomized, double-blind, crossover study with dexametha-
    sone in cancer patients receiving emetogenic chemotherapy. Ann Oncol 2 : 517–518
7. Arnold DJ, Ribiero V, Bulkin W (1980) Metoclopramide versus prochlorperazine in
    the prevention of vomiting from diamminedichloroplatinum (abstract). Proc Clin
    Oncol 21 : 344
8. Basurto C, Roila F, Bracardi S, Tonato M, Ballatori E, Del Favero A (1988) A double-
    blind trial comparing antiemetic efficacy and toxicity of metoclopramide versus me-
    thylprednisolone versus domperidone in patients receiving doxorubicin chemother-
    apy alone or in combination with other antiblastic agents. Am J Clin Oncol 11 :
    594–596
9. Belt RJ, Rhodes J, Taylor S (1981) Antiemetic therapy for patients receiving cisdiam-
    minedichloroplatinum(II): a randomized, double-blind study comparing metoclo-
    pramide and prochlorperazine. In: Poster DS, Penta JS, Bruno S, (eds) Treatment of
    cancer chemotherapy-induced nausea and vomiting. Masson, New York, pp 153–158
10. Bennett JM, Byrne P, Desai A et al (1985) A randomized multicenter trial for
    cyclophosphamide, Novantrone and 5-fluorouracil (CNF) versus cyclophosphamide,
    Adriamycin and 5-fluorouracil (CAF) in patients with metastatic breast cancer. Invest
    New Drugs 3 : 179–185
11. Bleiberg H, Piccart M, Lips S, Panzer JM, N'Koua Mbon JB (1992) A phase I trial of a
    new antiemetic drug – clebopride malate – in cisplatin-treated patients. Ann Oncol
    3 : 141–143
12. Bloom BS (1989) Risk and cost of gastrointestinal side effects associated with non-
    steroidal anti-inflammatory drugs. Arch Intern Med 149 : 1019–1022
13. Bonneterre J, Chevallier B, Metz R et al (1990) A randomized double-blind compari-
    son of ondansetron and metoclopramide in the prophylaxis of emesis induced by
    cyclophosphamide, fluorouracil, and doxorubicin or epirubicin chemotherapy. J Clin
    Oncol 8 : 1063–1069
14. Bregni M, Siena S, Di Nicola M, Bonadonna G, Gianni AM (1991) Tropisetron plus ha-
    loperidol to ameliorate nausea and vomiting associated with high-dose alkylating
    agent cancer chemotherapy. Eur J Cancer 27 : 561–565
15. Campbell M, Bateman DN (1992) Pharmacokinetic optimisation of antiemetic thera-
    py. Clin Pharmacokinet 23 : 147–160
16. Carr BI, Blayney DW, Goldberg A, Braly P, Metter GE, Doroshow JH (1987) High
    doses of prochlorperazine for cisplatin-induced emesis. A prospective, random,
    dose–response study. Cancer 60 : 2165–2169
17. Cassileth PA, Lusk EJ, Torri S, DiNubile N, Gerson SL (1983) Antiemetic efficacy of de-
    xamethasone therapy in patients receiving cancer chemotherapy. Arch Int Med 43 :
    1347–1349
18. Cersosimo RJ, Bromer R, Hoffer S, Welch J, Abrahamson M, Ki Hong W (1985) The an-
    tiemetic activity of droperidol administered by intramuscular injection during cis-
    platin chemotherapy: a pilot study. Drug Intell Clin Pharmacol 19 : 118–121
19. Chevallier B, Cappelaere P, Splinter T et al (1997) A double-blind, multicentre compa-
    rison of intravenous dolasetron mesilate and metoclopramide in the prevention of
    nausea and vomiting in cancer patients receiving high-dose cisplatin chemotherapy.
    Support Care Cancer 5 : 22–30
20. Chiara S, Campora E, Lionetto R, Bruzzi P, Rosso R (1987) Methylprednisolone for the
    control of CMF-induced emesis. Am J Clin Oncol 10 : 264–267
21. Clavel M, Bolot JE, Philippe-Bert J, Putot JP, Rodary C, Pommatau E (1978) Essai com-
    paratif en double insu de deux doses i.v. (50 mg et 10 mg) de metopimazine (1) dans

la prevention de nausées et des vomissements de la chimiotherapie anticancéreuse. Lyon Med 239 : 307–309

22. Colls BM, Ferry PG, Gray AJ, Harvey VJ, McQueen EG (1980) The antiemetic activity of tetrahydrocannabinol versus metoclopramide and thiethylperazine in patients undergoing cancer chemotherapy. N Z Med J 91 : 449–451

23. Cox R, Newman CE, Leyland MJ (1982) Metoclopramide in the reduction of nausea and vomiting associated with combined chemotherapy. Cancer Chemother Pharmacol 8 : 133–135

24. Cunningham D, Soukop M, Gilchrist NL et al (1985) Randomised trial of intravenous high dose metoclopramide and intramuscular chlorpromazine in controlling nausea and vomiting induced by cytotoxic drugs. BMJ 290 : 604–605

25. Cunningham D, Evans C, Gazet J-C et al (1987) Comparison of antiemetic efficacy of domperidone, metoclopramide, and dexamethasone in patients receiving outpatient chemotherapy regimens. BMJ 295 : 256

26. Cunningham D, Bradley CJ, Forrest GJ et al (1988) A randomized trial of oral nabilone and prochlorperazine compared to intravenous metoclopramide and dexamethasone in the treatment of nausea and vomiting induced by chemotherapy regimens containing cisplatin or cisplatin analogues. Eur J Cancer Clin Oncol 24 : 686–689

27. Cunningham D, Turner A, Hawthorn J et al (1989) Ondansetron with and without dexamethasone to treat chemotherapy-induced emesis. Lancet I : 1323

28. Lebeau B, Depierre A, Giovanni M et al (1996) The efficacy of a combination of ondansetron, methylprednisolone and metopimazine in patients previously uncontrolled with a dual antiemetic treatment in cisplatin-based chemotherapy. Ann Oncol 8 : 887–892

29. De Wit R, Schmitz PIM, Verweij J et al (1996) Analysis of cumulative probabilities shows that the efficacy of 5-HT_3 antagonist prophylaxis is not maintained. J Clin Oncol 14 : 644–651

30. Drapkin RL, Sokl GH, Paladine WJ, Polackwich R, Lyman G et al (1982) The antiemetic effect and dose response of dexamethasone in patients receiving cis-platinum (abstract). Proc Am Soc Clin Oncol 1 : 64

31. D'Souza DP, Reyntjens A, Thomas RD (1980) Domperidone in the prevention of nausea and vomiting induced by antineoplastic agents: a three-fold evaluation. Curr Ther Res 27 : 384–390

32. DuBois A, Vach W, Wechsel U, et al (1996) 5-Hydroxyindole-acetic acid and cortisol excretion as predictors of chemotherapy-induced emesis. Br J Cancer 74 : 1137–1140

33. Ekert H, Waters KD, Jurk IH, Mobilia J, Loughnan P (1979) Ameloration of cancer chemotherapy-induced nausea and vomiting by delta-9-tetrahydrocannabinol. Med J Aust 2 : 657–659

34. Fauser AA, Bleiberg H, Chevallier B et al (1996) A double-blind, randomized, parallel study of IV dolasetron mesilate versus IV metoclopramide in patients receiving moderately emetogenic chemotherapy. Cancer J 9 : 196–202

35. Fredrikson M, Hursti T, Fårst CJ et al (1992) Nausea in cancer chemotherapy is inversely related to urinary cortisol excretion. Br J Cancer 65 : 779–780

36. Frytak S, Moertel CG, O'Fallon JR et al (1979) Delta-9-tetrahydrocannabinol as an antiemetic for patients receiving cancer chemotherapy. Ann Intern Med 91 : 825–830

37. Frytak S, Moertel CG, Eagan RT, O'Fallon JR (1981) A double-blind comparison of metoclopramide and prochlorperazine as antiemetics for platinum therapy (abstract). Proc Am Soc Clin Oncol 22 : 421

38. Gercovich FG, Nahmod VE, Pirola CJ, Morgenfeld EL, Rivarola EJ (1984) A double-blind randomized, cross-over study comparing domperidone to metoclopramide as

antiemetic prevention in cancer chemotherapy (abstract). Proc Am Soc Clin Oncol 3 : 89

39. Goldstein D, Levi JA, Woods RL, Russel J, Morgan J, Kerestes Z (1989) Double-blind randomized cross-over trial of dexamethasone and prochlorperazine as anti-emetics for cancer chemotherapy. Oncology 46 : 105–108

40. Gordon CJ, Pazdur R, Zicarelli A, Cummings G, Al-Sarraf M (1989) Metoclopramide versus metoclopramide and lorazepam: superiority of combined therapy in the control of cisplatin-induced emesis. Cancer 63 : 578–582

41. Gralla RJ, Itri L, Pisko S, et al (1981) Antiemetic efficacy of high-dose metoclopramide: randomized trials with placebo and prochlorperazine in patients with chemotherapy-induced vomiting. N Engl J Med 305 : 905–909

42. Greenberg DB, Surman OS, Clarke J, Baer L (1987) Alprazolam for phobic nausea and vomiting related to cancer chemotherapy. Cancer Treat Rep 71 : 549–560

43. Grossman B, Lessin LS, Cohen P (1979) Droperidol prevents nausea and vomiting from cis-platinum. N Engl J Med 301 : 47

44. Grunberg SM (1993) Potential for combination therapy with the new antiserotonergic agents. Eur J Cancer [A] 29 [Suppl 1] : S39–S41

45. Grunberg SM, Gala KV, Lampenfeld M et al (1984) Comparison of the antiemetic effect of high-dose intravenous metoclopramide and high-dose intravenous haloperidol in a randomized double-blind crossover study. J Clin Oncol 2 : 782–787

46. Grunberg SM, Akerley WL, Krailo MD, Johnson KB, Baker CR, Cariffe PA (1986) Comparison of metoclopramide and metoclopramide plus dexamethasone for complete protection from cisplatin-induced emesis. Cancer Invest 4 : 379–385

47. Grunewald HW, Rosner F (1984) Dexamethasone as an antiemetic during cancer chemotherapy. Ann Intern Med 101 : 398

48. Haid M (1984) Steroid antiemesis may be harmful. N Engl J Med 304 : 1237

49. Hamik A, Peroutka SJ (1989) Differential interactions of traditional and novel antiemetics with dopamine D_2 and 5-hydroxytryptamine$_3$ receptors. Cancer Chemother Pharmacol 2 : 307–310

50. Harris AL (1982) Cytotoxic-therapy-induced vomiting is mediated via enkephalin pathways. Lancet I : 714

51. Herman TS, Einhorn LH, Jones SE et al (1979) Superiority of nabilone over prochlorperazine as an antiemetic in patients receiving cancer chemotherapy. N Engl J Med 300 : 1295–1297

52. Herrstedt J, Hannibal J, Hallas J, Andersen E, Lauersen LC, Hansen M (1991) High-dose metoclopramide+lorazepam versus low-dose metoclopramide+lorazepam+dehydrobenzperidol in the treatment of cisplatin-induced nausea and vomiting. Ann Oncol 2 : 223–227

53. Herrstedt J, Hyttel J, Pedersen J (1993) Interaction of the antiemetic metopimazine and anticancer agents with brain dopamine D_2, 5-hydroxytryptamine$_3$, histamine H1, muscarine cholinergic and α-1 adrenergic receptors. Cancer Chemother Pharmacol 33 : 53–56

54. Herrstedt J, Sigsgaard T, Boesgaard M, Jensen TP, Dombernowsky P (1993) Ondansetron plus metopimazine compared with ondansetron alone in patients receiving moderately emetogenic chemotherapy. N Engl J Med 328 : 1076–1080

55. Herrstedt J, Sigsgaard T, Angelo HR, Kampmann JP, Hansen M (1997) Dose-finding study of oral metopimazine. Support Care Cancer 5 : 38–43

56. Herrstedt J, Sigsgaard T, Handberg J, Schousboe BMB, Hansen M, Dombernowsky P (1997) Randomized, double-blind comparison of ondansetron versus ondansetron

plus metopimazine as antiemetic prophylaxis during platinum-based chemotherapy. J Clin Oncol 15 : 1690–1696

57. Hesketh PJ, Gandara DR, Hainsworth J, Edelman M, Webber LM, McManus M (1996) Addition of the dopamine D_2 antagonist prochlorperazine to granisetron/dexamethasone: improved control of acute emesis from high dose cisplatin (abstract). Proc Am Soc Clin Oncol 15 : 540

58. Homesley HD, Gainey JM, Jobson VN et al (1982) Double-blind placebo-controlled study of metoclopramide in cisplatin-induced emesis. N Engl J Med 307 : 250–251

59. Hursti TJ, Fredrikson M, Steineck G et al (1993) Endogenous cortisol exerts antiemetic effect similar to that of exogenous corticosteroids. Br J Cancer 68 : 112–114

60. Israel L, Rodary C (1978) Treatment of nausea and vomiting related to anticancerous multiple combination chemotherapy: results of two controlled studies. J Int Med Res 6 : 235–240

61. Italian Group for Antiemetic Research (1995) Dexamethasone, granisetron, or both for the prevention of nausea and vomiting during chemotherapy for cancer. N Engl J Med 332 : 1–5

62. Jones AL, Hill AS, Soukop M et al (1991) Comparison of dexamethasone and ondansetron in the prophylaxis of emesis induced by moderately emetogenic chemotherapy. Lancet 338 : 483–487

63. Joss RA, Galeazzi RL, Bischoff AK, Pirovino M, Ryssel HJ, Brunner KW (1986) The antiemetic activity of high-dose alizapride and high-dose metoclopramide in patients receiving cancer chemotherapy: a prospective randomized, double-blind trial. Clin Pharmacol Ther 39 : 619–624

64. Kaasa S, Kvaløy S, Dicato M et al (1990) A comparison of ondansetron with metoclopramide in the prophylaxis of chemotherapy-induced nausea and vomiting: a randomized, double-blind study. Eur J Cancer 26 : 311–314

65. Kahn T, Elias EG, Mason GR (1978) A single dose of metoclopramide in the control of vomiting from cis-dichlorodiammineplatinum(II) in man. Cancer Treat Rep 62 : 1106–1107

66. Kelley SL, Braun TJ, Meyer TJ, Rempel P, Pearlman NW (1986) Trial of droperidol as an antiemetic in cisplatin chemotherapy. Cancer Treat Rep 70 : 469–472

67. Kessler JF, Alberts DS, Aapro MS et al (1986) An effective five-drug antiemetic combination for prevention of chemotherapy-related nausea and vomiting. Experience in eighty-four patients. Cancer Chemother Pharmacol 12 : 282–286

68. Koval E, Garay G (1983) Metoclopramide or domperidone in the prevention of chemotherapy-induced nausea and vomiting (abstract). Second European Conference on Clinical Oncology, November 1983, Amsterdam, A23-03

69. Kris MG, Gralla RJ, Tyson LB, et al (1985) Improved control of cisplatin-induced emesis with high-dose metoclopramide and with combinations of metoclopramide, dexamethasone, and diphenhydramine. Cancer 55 : 527–534

70. Kris MG, Gralla RJ, Clark RA, Tyson LB, Groshen S (1987) Antiemetic control and prevention of side effects of anticancer therapy with lorazepam or diphenhydramine when used in combination with metoclopramide plus dexamethasone. Cancer 60 : 2816–2822

71. Kris MG, Gralla RJ, Tyson LB, Clark RA, Cirrincione C, Groshen S (1989) Controlling delayed vomiting: double-blind, randomized trial comparing placebo, dexamethasone alone, and metoclopramide plus dexamethasone in patients receiving cisplatin. J Clin Oncol 7 : 108–114

72. Lane M, Vogel CL, Ferguson J et al (1991) Dronabinol and prochlorperazine in combination for treatment of cancer chemotherapy-induced nausea and vomiting. J Pain Symptom Manage 6 : 352–359

73. Lee C-W, Suh C-W, Lee J-S et al (1994) Ondansetron compared with ondansetron plus metoclopramide in the prevention of cisplatin-induced emesis. J Korean Med Sci 9 : 369–375

74. Levitt M, Sharma RN, Faiman C et al (1979) Normal metyrapone response after 1 month of high-dose methylprednisolone in cancer patients: a phase I study. Cancer Treat Rep 63 : 1327–1330

75. Livera P, Trojano M, Simone IL et al (1985) Acute changes in blood CSF barrier permselectivity to serum proteins after intrathecal methotrexate and CNS irradiation. J Neurol 231 : 336–339

76. Longo DL, Wesley M, Howser D, Hubbard SM, Anderson T, Young RC (1982) Results of a randomized, double-blind crossover trial of scopolamine versus placebo administered by transdermal patch for the control of cisplatin-induced emesis. Cancer Treat Rep 66 : 1975–1976

77. Marini G, Murray S, Goldhirsch A et al (1996) The effect of adjuvant prednisone combined with CMF on patterns of relapse and occurrence of second malignancies in patients with breast cancer. Ann Oncol 7 : 245–250

78. Markman M, Sheidler V, Ettinger DS, Quaskey SA, Mellits EA (1984) Antiemetic efficacy of dexamethasone. Randomized, double-blind, crossover study with prochlorperazine in patients receiving cancer chemotherapy. N Engl J Med 311 : 549–552

79. Marschner NW, Adler M, Nagel GA, Christmann D, Fenzl E, Upadhyaya B (1991) Double-blind randomised trial of the antiemetic efficacy and safety of ondansetron and metoclopramide in advanced breast cancer patients treated with epirubicin and cyclophosphamide. Eur J Cancer 27 : 1137–1140

80. Marty M, Pouillart P, Scholl S et al (1990) Comparison of the 5-hydroxytryptamine$_3$ antagonist ondansetron (GR 38032F) with high dose metoclopramide in the control of cisplatin-induced emesis. N Engl J Med 322 : 816–821

81. Matsumoto I, Aikawa T, Kanda T et al (1989) Amelioration of cisplatin-induced vomiting and anorexia by methylprednisolone. Gan To Kagaku Ryoko 16 : 833–838

82. Meden H, Meissner O, Conrad A, Kuhn W (1996) Improved control of nausea and emesis with a new bromazepam-containing ondansetron regimen in ovarian cancer patients receiving chemotherapy with carboplatin and cyclophosphamide. Eur J Gynaecol Oncol 17 : 114–122

83. Mellink WA, Blijham GH, Van Deyk WA (1984) Amitriptyline plus fluphenazine to prevent chemotherapy-induced emesis in cancer patients: a double-blind randomized cross-over study. Eur J Cancer Clin Oncol 20 : 1147–1150

84. Meyer BR, O'Mara V, Reidenberg MM (1987) A controlled clinical trial of the addition of transdermal scopolamine to a standard metoclopramide and dexamethasone antiemetic regimen. J Clin Oncol 5 : 1994–1997

85. Miner WD, Sanger GJ (1986) Inhibition of cisplatin-induced vomiting by selective 5-hydroxytryptamine M-receptor antagonism. Br J Pharmacol 88 : 497–499

86. Moertel CG, Reitemeier RJ (1969) Controlled clinical studies of orally administered antiemetic drugs. Gastroenterology 56 : 262–268

87. Moertel CG, Reitemeier RJ (1973) Controlled studies of metopimazine for the treatment of nausea and vomiting. J Clin Pharmacol 13 : 283–287

88. Moertel CG, Reitemeier RJ, Gage RP (1963) A controlled clinical evaluation of antiemetic drugs. JAMA 186 : 116–118

89. Moreno I, Rosell R, Abad A et al (1992) Comparison of three protracted antiemetic regimens for the control of delayed emesis in cisplatin-treated patients. Eur J Cancer [A] 28 : 1344–1347

90. Morran C, Smith DC, Anderson DA, McArdle CS (1979) Incidence of nausea and vomiting with cytotoxic chemotherapy: a prospective randomised trial of antiemetics. BMJ 19 : 1323–1324

91. Neidhart JA, Gagen M, Young D, Wilson HE (1981) Specific antiemetics for specific cancer chemotherapeutic agents: haloperidol versus benzquinamide. Cancer 47 : 1439–1443

92. Olver IN, Webster LK, Bishop JF, Clarke J, Hillcoat BL (1989) A dose finding study of prochlorperazine as an antiemetic for cancer chemotherapy. Eur J Cancer Clin Oncol 25 : 1457–1461

93. Olver IN, Wolf M, Laidlaw C et al (1992) A randomised double-blind study of high-dose intravenous prochlorperazine versus high-dose metoclopramide as antiemetics for cancer chemotherapy. Eur J Cancer [A] 28 : 1798–1802

94. Onsrud M, Moxnes A, Sollien A et al (1988) High-dose versus low-dose metoclopramide in the prevention of cisplatin-induced emesis. Cancer 61 : 2429–2432

95. Orr LE, McKerman JF, Bloome B (1980) Antiemetic effect of tetrahydrocannabinol compared with placebo and prochlorperazine in chemotherapy-associated nausea and vomiting. Arch Intern Med 140 : 1431–1433

96. Plasse TF, Gorter RW, Krasnow SH, Lane M, Shepard KV, Wadleigh RG (1991) Recent clinical experience with dronabinol. Pharmacol Biochem Behav 40 : 695–700

97. Pollera CF, Nardi M, Marolla P, Pinnaro P, Terzoli E, Giannarelli D (1989) Effective control of CMF-related emesis with high-dose dexamethasone: results of a double-blind crossover trial with metoclopramide and placebo. Am J Clin Oncol 12 : 524–529

98. Pollera CF, Nardi M, Marolla P, Calabresi F (1991) Alizapride alone or alizapride-dexamethasone compared with metoclopramide-dexamethasone in patients at high risk of acute emesis after cisplatin. Acta Oncol 30 : 725–729

99. Powell CB, Mutch DG, Ming-Shian K et al (1990) Dexamethasone used as an antiemetic in chemotherapy protocols inhibits natural cytotoxic cell activity. Cancer 65 : 466–472

100. Roila F, Tonato M, Basurto C et al (1987) Antiemetic activity of high doses of metoclopramide combined with methylprednisolone versus metoclopramide alone in cisplatin-treated cancer patients: a randomized double-blind trial of the Italian Oncology Group for Clinical Research. J Clin Oncol 5 : 141–149

101. Roila F, Tonato M, Basurto C, Minotti V, Ballatori E, Del Favero A (1987) Double-blind controlled trial of the antiemetic efficacy and toxicity of methylprednisolone (MP), metoclopramide (MTC) and domperidone (DMP) in breast cancer patients treated with i.v. CMF. Eur J Cancer Clin Oncol 23 : 615–617

102. Roila F, Basurto C, Minotti V et al (1988) Methylprednisolone versus metoclopramide for prevention of nausea and vomiting in breast cancer patients treated with cyclophosphamide, methotrexate and 5-fluorouracil: a double-blind randomized study. Oncology 45 : 346–349

103. Roila F, Tonato M, Ballatori E, Del Favero A (1996) Comparative studies of various antiemetic regimens. Support Care Cancer 4 : 270–280

104. Rudd JA, Bunce KT, Naylor RJ (1996) The interaction of dexamethasone with ondansetron on drug-induced emesis in the ferret. Neuropharmacology 35 : 91–97

105. Sallan SE, Cronin C, Zelen M, Zinberg NE (1980) Antiemetics in patients receiving chemotherapy for cancer. A randomized comparison of delta-9-tetrahydrocannabinol and prochlorperazine. N Engl J Med 302 : 135–138

106. Saller R, Hellenbrecht D, Hellstern A, Hess H (1985) Improved benefit/risk ratio of higher-dose metoclopramide therapy during cisplatin-induced emesis. Eur J Clin Pharmacol 29 : 311–312

107. Sherlock P, Hartmann WH (1962) Adrenal steroids and the pattern of metastases of breast cancer. JAMA 181 : 313–317

108. Stephen LC, Rine J et al (1981) The role of prostaglandins in the excessive nausea and vomiting after intravascular cis-platinum therapy. Gynecol Oncol 12 : 89–91

109. Swann IL, Thompson EN, Qureshi K (1979) Domperidone or metoclopramide in preventing chemotherapeutically induced nausea and vomiting. BMJ II : 1188–1189

110. Tsukuda M, Furukawa S, Kokatsu T, Enomoto H, Kubota A, Furukawa M (1995) Comparison of granisetron alone and granisetron plus hydroxyzine hydrochloride for prophylactic treatment of emesis induced by cisplatin chemotherapy. Eur J Cancer [A] 31 : 1647–1649

111. Vallejo C, Rabinovich M, Leone B, Gonzales J (1988) Toxicity and dose response of intravenous (I.V.) metopimazine (MTZ) as preventive of high-dose cisplatin (CDDP)-induced emesis (abstract). Proc Am Soc Clin Oncol 7 : 286

112. Warr D (1997) Standard treatment of chemotherapy-induced emesis. Support Care Cancer 5 : 12–16

113. Warr D, Willan A, Fine S et al (1991) Superiority of granisetron to dexamethasone plus prochlorperazine in the prevention of chemotherapy-induced emesis. J Natl Cancer Inst 83 : 1169–1173

114. Williams CJ, Bolton A, De Pemberton R, Whitehouse JMA (1980) Antiemetics for patients treated with antitumor chemotherapy. Cancer Clin Trials 3 : 363–367

115. Winokur SH, Baker JJ, Lokey JL, Price NA, Bowen J (1981) Dexamethasone in the treatment of nausea and vomiting from cancer chemotherapy. J Med Assoc Ga 70 : 263–264

116. Zambetti M, Bajetta E, Bidoli P, Verusio C (1985) Antiemetic activity of metoclopramide versus alizapride during cancer chemotherapy. Tumori 71 : 609–614

117. Zylberait D, Krulik M, Audebert AA, Debray J (1981) Essai comparatif de deux medicaments dans le traitement des vomissements induits par la chimiotherapie anti-cancéreuse. Semin Hopitaux 57 : 47

Optimal Selection of Antiemetics in Children Receiving Cancer Chemotherapy

Fausto Roila, Matti S. Aapro, Alan Stewart

ABSTRACT Only a few studies have been carried out specifically on the prevention of nausea and vomiting in children receiving chemotherapy. In these patients, older antiemetic drugs such as metoclopramide and phenothiazines had moderate efficacy and induced significant side effects, especially marked sedation and extrapyramidal reactions.

In comparative trials, the 5-HT$_3$ receptor antagonists have shown better efficacy and tolerability than chlorpromazine or metoclopramide combined with dexamethasone.

The combination of a 5-HT$_3$ receptor antagonist plus dexamethasone is superior to a 5-HT$_3$ receptor antagonist alone and should be the standard antiemetic prophylaxis in all pediatric patients receiving highly or moderately emetogenic chemotherapy.

The optimal dose and scheduling of these antiemetic drugs need to be studied, as well as the antiemetic efficacy, in the prevention of chemotherapy-induced delayed and anticipatory emesis in children.

Introduction

Nausea and vomiting, the most distressing side effects of adult cancer chemotherapy, are also a major problem in the treatment of childhood malignancies. They can lead to increased patient morbidity, e. g., electrolyte imbalance, dehydration, poor nutrition and prolonged hospitalization. Intensification of antineoplastic regimens, particularly with multi-day regimens, has exacerbated this problem. Good control of nausea and vomiting is mandatory in children receiving chemotherapy. Unfortunately, only a few studies have been carried out specifically in children on the prevention of these side effects. It is inappropriate to assume that results obtained in studies conducted in adult patients can be directly applied to children. Metabolism and side effects of drugs may be different in pediatric patients than in adults. This review will focus on the comparative studies in children published so far, but will not include studies that have evaluated antiemetics in children subjected to high-dose chemotherapy such as is used in bone marrow transplantation, which will be considered in another paper.

Before the Introduction of 5-HT$_3$ Receptor Antagonists

Before the introduction of the 5-HT$_3$ receptor antagonists, phenothiazines and metoclopramide were the most commonly prescribed antiemetics in pediatric oncology. It is well established that children are more susceptible than older patients to the extrapyramidal reactions induced by metoclopramide, and that these side effects are dose related. After the demonstration that high-dose intravenous metoclopramide was efficacious in the prevention of cisplatin-induced emesis in adult patients [15], dose-finding studies were carried out to identify the optimal intravenous (i.v.) dose in children [1, 13, 37]. In one of these, 26 children were randomized to one of four different doses of metoclopramide (0.25, 0.5, 1.0, and 2.0 mg/kg), administered every 3 h for five doses starting 30 min before chemotherapy [13]. All patients receiving doses higher than 1 mg/kg developed extrapyramidal reactions. Therefore, the dose of 0.5 mg/kg i.v. was suggested for subsequent comparative trials. In another pilot study carried out in eight children, the tolerability of one to three courses of metoclopramide at doses of 0.5–2 mg/kg i.v. every 4–8 h for up 48 h was evaluated [37]. Seven out of eight patients (88%) experienced a total of 13 extrapyramidal reactions (EPR), and seven of these 13 episodes occurred in patients receiving less than 1 mg/kg metoclopramide.

Finally, Allen [1] evaluated metoclopramide at nine increasing doses from 0.2 mg/kg to 3 mg/kg i.v. every 2 h for four doses with the addition of diphenhydramine for possible prevention of EPR (0.5 mg/kg i.v. with the first and third doses of metoclopramide). In 45 pediatric patients treated with cisplatin and cyclophosphamide, the toxicity was minimal with metoclopramide doses of less than 2 mg/kg, but with a metoclopramide dose exceeding 2 mg/kg, 15% of patients had extrapyramidal reactions and 33% had akathisia.

Three comparative studies of intravenous metoclopramide in the prevention of chemotherapy-induced nausea and vomiting in children have been published [14, 27, 36]. In a double-blind trial published by Graham-Pole, 50 children were randomly assigned to receive metoclopramide or chlorpromazine, both at 0.5 mg/kg per dose i.v. beginning 30 min before chemotherapy and repeated every 3 h for five doses [14]. Children treated with chlorpromazine had fewer emetic episodes (1.8) and a shorter duration of vomiting (4.2 h) than those treated with metoclopramide (3.5 episodes and 9.0 h, respectively). Furthermore, EPR were reported significantly more often for metoclopramide- (5/24, 21%) than for chlorpromazine-treated patients (1/26, 3.8%), but somnolence was much more frequently observed with chlorpromazine (53%).

Interestingly, the superiority of chlorpromazine over metoclopramide proved significant in boys but not in girls, in older but not in younger patients, in previously treated rather than previously untreated patients, and in those receiving predominantly alkylating agents but not in those receiving antimetabolites. Swann compared metoclopramide (0.5 mg/kg i.v.) with domperidone (up to 1 mg/kg i.v.) using an open crossover design in 18 children receiving chemotherapy for a variety of malignant diseases [36]. Domperidone was statistically superior to metoclopramide, with median numbers of emetic episodes of 0.5 and 4.0, respectively.

Finally, in a double-blind crossover study, a four-agent combination of metoclopramide (2 mg/kg i.v. every 2–6 h for four doses) plus benztropine to prevent EPR (0.04 mg/kg i.v. with the first and third doses of metoclopramide) and dexamethasone (0.7 mg/kg i.v.) and lorazepam (0.05 mg/kg p.o. every 12 h for two doses) was compared with chlorpromazine (0.825 mg/kg i.v. every 6 h for four doses) [27]. Marshall reported that the combination showed superior antiemetic efficacy over chlorpromazine alone, with a complete response in 46% and 19% of patients, respectively, and it was preferred by 77% of the patients. All children slept from late afternoon on the day of chemotherapy until the next morning. The incidence of moderately sedated children, the sedated state being defined as one requiring physical contact for the child to be awakened, was 27% with the metoclopramide combination and 35% with chlorpromazine. Dystonia was observed in only one patient treated with the combination (4%).

Phenothiazine compounds have antiemetic activity, and a double-blind study evaluated the antiemetic efficacy and tolerability of chlorpromazine (0.5 mg/kg single dose i.v.) compared with methylprednisolone (4 mg/kg single dose i.v.), both repeated after 6 h if patients vomited, in 20 children with previous experience of significant emesis with chemotherapy [28]. Similar results were shown in both arms, with 50% of patients obtaining a complete response in each arm and a mean number of 3.5 emetic episodes with chlorpromazine and 3.1 with methylprednisolone. Sedation was less common with the latter drug.

The positive results obtained with intravenous chlorpromazine in children in the two double-blind studies cited [14, 28] clearly contrast with those reported from an open study in which 23 children received intermittent antiemetic prophylaxis with phenothiazines (prochlorperazine suppositories 12.5–25 mg every 4-6 h or chlorpromazine 25–100 mg i.v. every 4–6 h) [39]. The intensity and duration of nausea and vomiting were significantly higher during courses with prophylactic phenothiazines. Therefore, it seemed that phenothiazines did not reduce children's nausea and vomiting and might even have been associated with an increase in symptoms.

There are a small number of reports on cannabinoids used as antiemetics in children. A double-blind crossover study reported by Ekert demonstrated that oral delta-9-tetrahydrocannabinol at a dose of 10 mg/m^2 2 h before and 4, 8, 16, and 24 h after chemotherapy was superior to oral prochlorperazine (5–10 mg) 2 h before and 8, 16, and 24 h after chemotherapy in 14 children and also superior to low-dose oral metoclopramide (5–10 mg p.o.) 2 h before and 8, 16 and 24 h after chemotherapy in 19 children [11]. Delta-9-tetrahydrocannabinol induced significantly more drowsiness and a "high" in two patients.

Nabilone, a synthetic cannabinoid, was used in two double-blind crossover studies in 18 and 30 children [7, 9] and in one open crossover study in nine children [32] at a dose of 0.5–2 mg p.o. two to three times a day. These trials showed superiority of nabilone over oral domperidone, 5–15 mg three times a day, and oral prochlorperazine, 5–10 mg two to three times a day. Nabilone was preferred by the patients, although it induced significantly more adverse events, such as dizziness, drowsiness, and mood changes, than the comparators. The adverse side effect profile means that these agents are no longer popular as antiemetics.

Many of the early trials of antiemetics in children were poorly designed and did not take into account the different emetogenic potency of the cytotoxic agents or the differences between acute and delayed emesis. Studies also included a mixture of pretreated and chemotherapy-naive children. Many of the trials recruited too few patients to permit robust statistical analysis. In summary, before the introduction of the 5-HT$_3$ receptor antagonists, only nine comparative studies using different antiemetics were reported, and reliable conclusions are difficult to make.

Metoclopramide at low standard doses seems inferior to chlorpromazine or domperidone. Chlorpromazine was as efficacious as methylprednisolone, but less sedation was induced by this latter drug. High-dose intravenous metoclopramide combined with benztropine, dexamethasone, and lorazepam was superior to chlorpromazine. Cannabinoids demonstrated better antiemetic efficacy than oral prochlorperazine, oral domperidone, or low doses of oral metoclopramide. They were preferred by the patients but were associated with unpleasant side effects.

Overall, these antiemetic drugs had moderate efficacy and induced significant side effects, especially marked sedation and EPR, in children undergoing cancer chemotherapy.

5-HT$_3$ Receptor Antagonists

Pilot Studies

The early studies with the 5-HT$_3$ receptor antagonist antiemetics have been of better design, and larger numbers of children have been recruited.

Ondansetron has been evaluated in three open multicenter European studies involving 429 children. The efficacy and tolerability of intravenous ondansetron, 5 mg/m^2 or 8 mg, followed by oral maintenance doses of 2, 4, or 8 mg depending on the body surface area, given every 8 h for 2 days after non-cisplatin chemotherapy or for 5 days after cisplatin chemotherapy, were evaluated by Jurgens [22]. Sixty-eight percent of all ondansetron treatment days were free of emesis. When the results were analyzed according to the most emetogenic agent given, 36%, 59%, and 75% of children reported fewer than three emetic episodes on their "worst day" during chemotherapy with cisplatin, ifosfamide, and other, less emetogenic agents, respectively. The incidence of adverse events was low, with headaches being the most frequently reported (4%). Similar results were reported in one of these three trials published singly [18].

In another open trial, ondansetron was given to 20 children with leukemia treated with combination chemotherapy including cyclophosphamide and cytarabine [5]. Ondansetron was administered at 3–5 mg/m^2 i.v. and 2, 3, or 4 mg p.o. every 8 h for a total of 14 doses, based on the children's body surface area, starting concurrently with the intravenous dose. Vomiting was recorded in only two of 20 patients on day 1 and in five of 20 patients on days 2–5. A further open study was carried out in 15 children receiving ondansetron at 5 mg/m^2 by i.v. infusion or 4-mg oral tablets every 8 h for 24 h [35]. Nausea and vomiting were completely controlled in 27 of the 38 courses of chemotherapy evaluated.

Panzarella treated 26 children undergoing highly or moderately emetogenic chemotherapy. Complete protection from vomiting was obtained in 42% with 0.15 mg/kg i.v. ondansetron followed by two oral doses of 4–8 mg [31]. Finally, 16 pediatric patients with acute lymphoblastic leukemia were studied during repeated cycles of chemotherapy, given with or without ondansetron (0.15 mg/kg i.v. before chemotherapy and 2–3 h after) [20]. Compared with chemotherapy given without any antiemetic, ondansetron completely protected patients during more than 55% of chemotherapy cycles, except for those in which cyclophosphamide was used.

Granisetron has been evaluated in three pilot studies [8, 21, 29]. In 30 children who were being treated with various anticancer drugs and who had previously had poor control of emesis, 20 µg/kg i.v granisetron. induced complete protection in 39% of chemotherapy courses [21].

Craft studied 40 children receiving various anticancer drugs. A single 40-μg/kg dose of granisetron i.v. induced complete protection from vomiting and nausea in 27.5% of patients [8].

Finally, 22 children who had experienced emesis in the previous course of chemotherapy, when they received metoclopramide and promethazine as antiemetic prophylaxis, received 40 μg/kg granisetron i.v. as a single dose in the subsequent course [29]. A complete response was obtained in 59.1% of these previously refractory patients.

Tropisetron was used in 131 children treated with a range of anticancer drugs. A single i.v. injection of 0.2 mg/kg tropisetron (maximum 5 mg) induced complete protection from acute vomiting and nausea in 67% of children [3].

In 19 children with previous experience of emesis related to chemotherapy, 0.2 mg/kg tropisetron i.v. (maximum 5 mg) induced complete protection from emesis in 77% of 169 chemotherapy courses [16]. Cefalo studied 15 children with emesis refractory to metoclopramide-based regimens during previous chemotherapy. No more than two emetic episodes were observed in 118 of 184 (64%) treatment days with 2 or 5 mg tropisetron i.v. [6].

In two other studies, in each of which 15 patients were enrolled, who were treated with cisplatin or moderately emetogenic drugs, 5 mg/m^2 tropisetron i.v. (maximum 5 mg) induced complete protection from acute nausea and vomiting in 53.3% and 68.7% of children, respectively [4, 12]. Finally, in ten patients with previous experience of emesis refractory to hydroxyzine, 5 mg tropisetron i.v. or p.o. induced complete protection from vomiting in 14 out of 20 (70%) chemotherapy cycles [33].

In conclusion, many pilot studies of 5-HT$_3$ receptor antagonists have shown good antiemetic efficacy and very low toxicity in the pediatric chemotherapy field.

Dose-Finding Studies in Children

The optimal dose of three of the 5-HT$_3$ receptor antagonists for use in children has been evaluated in five trials. Two dose-finding studies have been carried out with granisetron. One double-blind study in 80 children showed that the mean number of vomiting episodes and the percentage of patients who had one or fewer emetic episodes was lower with the 40 μg/kg i.v. single dose (one episode and 56% protection rate) than with the 10 μg/kg (two episodes and 48.3%) or the 20 μg/kg i.v. dose (three episodes and 42.0%). This difference was not, however, statistically significant [24].

In the other open study, doses of 20 and 40 μg/kg i.v. seem superior to 10 μg/kg i.v. [26]. In fact, in 24 children submitted to highly or moderately emetogenic chemotherapy, complete protection from nausea and vomiting was obtained in two of eight patients with 10 µg/kg and in five of eight patients each with 20 µg/kg and 40 µg/kg.

In a dose-finding study with tropisetron, Suarez showed that a dose of 0.20 mg/kg i.v. was significantly more efficacious in preventing vomiting than lower doses (0.05 and 0.10 mg/kg i.v.) or placebo [34].

Recently, two open studies have evaluated the optimal intravenous and oral dose of dolasetron for children submitted to moderately or highly emetogenic chemotherapy [25, 38]. In the first study with 46 enrolled patients, four different single i.v. doses (0.6, 1.2, 1.8, and 2.4 mg/kg) were administered before chemotherapy was evaluated. Complete responses were obtained in 10%, 25%, 66.7%, and 33.3% of patients, respectively. Headache, which was the commonest side effect, was reported by 13% of children. The dose of 1.8 mg/kg was suggested for further studies [25]. In 32 patients, a single oral dose of dolasetron of 0.6, 1.2, and 1.8 mg/kg administered before chemotherapy was evaluated. A complete response was obtained in 33.3%, 30.8%, and 50.0% of patients, respectively, confirming that the 1.8 mg/kg oral dose appears to be the most effective dose of dolasetron [38].

Although indicative, these studies are small and insufficient to identify the absolute optimal oral and intravenous doses of the 5-HT$_3$ receptor antagonists in children.

Comparative Studies

Only four studies have compared the 5-HT$_3$ receptor antagonists with older antiemetic drugs in the pediatric population [2, 10, 17, 19].

In one open study, intravenous ondansetron (3 mg/m^2 or 8 mg, according to body surface area, repeated every 12 h) was compared with a combination, given i.v., of low-dose metoclopramide (10 mg/m^2 every 6 h) with procyclidine to decrease extrapyramidal reactions, plus dexamethasone (4 mg/m^2 followed by 2 mg/m^2 every 8 h) in 30 children receiving chemotherapy with daunorubicin, etoposide, cytarabine, and thioguanine [10]. Ondansetron showed superior antiemetic activity to the combination, with complete or major response being obtained in 93% and 33% of patients, respectively.

A similar study carried out in 88 children treated with ifosfamide-containing chemotherapy compared granisetron (20 µg/kg i.v.) with a combination, also given i.v., of chlorpromazine (0.3–0.5 mg/kg every 4–6 h) plus dexamethasone (2 mg/m^2 every 8 h) [17]. Granisetron was significantly superior to the chlorpromazine plus dexamethasone combination, with zero or one emetic episode observed in 51% versus 21% of patients, respectively. Granisetron induced less sedation, and EPR occurred in two patients receiving chlorpromazine and dexamethasone.

A double-blind study compared ondansetron (0.15 mg/kg i.v. for three doses) alone with the same ondansetron schedule combined with dexamethasone (8 mg/m^2 i.v. followed by 4–8 mg/m^2 i.v. every 4–6 h) in 33 patients receiving cisplatin, carboplatin, cyclophosphamide or ifosfamide. The combination of ondansetron plus dexamethasone was significantly superior to ondansetron alone, with complete protection from vomiting obtained by 61% and 23% of children, respectively [2].

Finally, Hirota from Japan reported an open crossover trial comparing granisetron (40 µg/kg i.v.) combined with methylprednisolone (10 mg/kg i.v.) with granisetron alone at the same dose in 20 children submitted to chemotherapy [19]. Complete control of vomiting was achieved in 19 of 20 (95%) patients receiving the combination and in 17 of the 20 (85%) treated with granisetron alone.

No comparative studies of different 5-HT$_3$ receptor antagonists have been reported in the pediatric population.

In conclusion, only a few well-designed studies comparing the 5-HT$_3$ receptor antagonists with older antiemetic drugs have been carried out. Ondansetron and granisetron have been shown to be superior to chlorpromazine or metoclopramide combined with dexamethasone. Furthermore, the 5-HT$_3$ receptor antagonists are less toxic. As in the adult population, the combination of a 5-HT$_3$ receptor antagonist and dexamethasone is superior to a 5-HT$_3$ receptor antagonist alone.

Issues Still to be Resolved

Because so few studies have been carried out in children, many problems remain unsolved. We cannot assume that children will respond to cytotoxic drugs or antiemetic agents in the same manner as adults. It has not been established whether all children receiving chemotherapy, even of low emetogenic potential, should receive antiemetic prophylaxis. Furthermore, we have little firm data on patient-related prognostic factors in children. From preliminary studies it seems that older children and girls might experience more chemotherapy-induced nausea and vomiting than infants and boys [23]. Finally, studies need to be undertaken to evaluate the incidence and optimal treatment of delayed and anticipatory emesis in children.

Consensus Statement

Recently, Ninane published guidelines for the use of antiemetics in children based on a survey conducted among the attending physicians of the hematology/oncology division of an American children's hospital. The survey showed wide variations in the indications for the use of ondansetron and the schedule of administration [30]. Unfortunately, these guidelines were based more on subjective opinions than on the results of clinical trials and are therefore of limited value. From the published data available, consensus can be achieved on the following points:

1. Guidelines for the use of antiemetics in children should be obtained from prospective randomized trials carried out in children rather than by extrapolation from adult studies.

   Degree of consensus   High
   Degree of confidence   Not applicable

2. All pediatric patients receiving highly or moderately emetogenic chemotherapy should receive antiemetic prophylaxis.

   Degree of consensus   High
   Degree of confidence   High

3. Phenothiazines and metoclopramide should not be used as first-line therapy due to their adverse side effect profile.

   Degree of consensus   High
   Degree of confidence   Medium

4. In these patients, a combination of a 5-HT$_3$ receptor antagonist plus dexamethasone should be the standard preventive antiemetic treatment.

   Degree of consensus   High
   Degree of confidence   Medium

5. The optimal dose and scheduling of the 5-HT$_3$ receptor antagonists have not been well studied, and more large, well-conducted trials are needed. At the present time a milligram per kilogram dose, similar to that used in adult patients, should be utilized in clinical practice.

   Degree of consensus   High
   Degree of confidence   Not available

6. No studies have specifically evaluated antiemetic drugs in the prevention of chemotherapy-induced delayed and anticipatory emesis in the pediatric population. Such studies need to be carried out.

   Degree of consensus   High
   Degree of confidence   Not applicable

References

1. Allen JC, Gralla R, Reilly L, Kellick M, Young C (1985) Metoclopramide: dose-related toxicity and preliminary antiemetic studies in children receiving cancer chemotherapy. J Clin Oncol 3 : 1136–1141
2. Alvarez O, Freeman A, Bedros A, Call SK, Volsch J, Kalbermatter O, Halverson J, Convoy L, Cook L, Mick K, Zimmerman G (1995) Randomized double-blind

crossover ondansetron-dexamethasone versus ondansetron-placebo study for the treatment of chemotherapy-induced nausea and vomiting in paediatric patients with malignancies. J Pediatr Hematol Oncol 17 : 145–150

3. Benoit Y, Hulstaert F, Vermylen C, Sariban E, Hoyoux C, Uyttebroeck A, Otten J, Laureys C, De Kerpel I, Nortier D, Ritter L, De Keyser P (1995) Tropisetron in the prevention of nausea and vomiting in 131 children receiving cytotoxic chemotherapy. Med Pediatr Oncol 25 : 457–462

4. Berberoglu S (1995) Prevention of emesis by tropisetron in children receiving combined chemotherapy with cisplatin. Pediatr Hematol Oncol 12 : 479–483

5. Carden PA, Mitchell SL, Waters KD, Tiedemann K, Ekert H (1990) Prevention of cyclophosphamide/cytarabine-induced emesis with ondansetron in children with leukaemia. J Clin Oncol 8 : 1531–1535

6. Cefalo G, Rottoli L, Armiraglio A, Pagan MG (1994) Tropisetron (ICS 205-930) in paediatric oncology: first results in patients refractory to antiemetic metoclopramide-based treatments. Am J Pediatr Hematol Oncol 16 : 242–245

7. Chan HSL, MacLeod SM, Correia JA (1987) Nabilone versus prochlorperazine for control of cancer chemotherapy-induced emesis in children: a double-blind, crossover trial. Paediatrics 79 : 946–952

8. Craft AW, Price L, Eden OB, Shaw P, Campbell R, Pierce DM, Murdoch R, Upward J (1995) Granisetron as antiemetic therapy in children with cancer. Med Pediatr Oncol 25 : 28–32

9. Dalzell AM, Bartlett H, Lilleyman JS (1986) Nabilone: an alternative antiemetic for cancer chemotherapy. Arch Dis Child 61 : 502–505

10. Dick GS, Meller ST, Pinkerton CR (1995) Randomised comparison of ondansetron and metoclopramide plus dexamethasone for chemotherapy induced emesis. Arch Dis Child 73 : 243–245

11. Ekert H, Waters KD, Jurg IH, Mobilia J, Loughnan P (1979) Amelioration of cancer chemotherapy-induced nausea and vomiting by delta-9-tetrahydrocannabinol. Med J Aust 2 : 657–659

12. Gershanovich M, Kolygin B, Pirgach N (1993) Tropisetron in the control of nausea and vomiting induced by combined cancer chemotherapy in children. Ann Oncol 4 [Suppl 3] : 35–37

13. Graham-Pole J, Engel S (1984) Dose-related extrapyramidal effect of metoclopramide in children receiving chemotherapy. Proc Am Soc Clin Oncol 3 : 104

14. Graham-Pole J, Weare J, Engel S, Gardner R, Metha P, Gross S (1986) Antiemetics in children receiving cancer chemotherapy: a double-blind prospective randomised study of metoclopramide with chlorpromazine. J Clin Oncol 4 : 1110–1113

15. Gralla RJ, Itri LM, Pisko SE, Squillante AE, Kelsen DP, Braun DW, Bordin LA, Braun TJ, Young CW (1981) Antiemetic efficacy of high-dose metoclopramide: randomised trials with placebo and prochlorperazine in patients with chemotherapy-induced nausea and vomiting. N Engl J Med 305 : 905–909

16. Hachimi-Idrissi S, De Schepper J, Maurus R, Otten J (1993) Prevention of emesis by ICS 205-930 in children receiving cytotoxic chemotherapy. Eur J Cancer 29A : 854–856

17. Hählen K, Quintana E, Pinkerton CR, Cedar E (1995) A randomised comparison of intravenously administered granisetron versus chlorpromazine plus dexamethasone in the prevention of ifosfamide-induced emesis in children. J Pediatr 126 : 309–313

18. Hewitt M, McQuade B, Stevens R (1993) The efficacy and safety of ondansetron in the prophylaxis of cancer-chemotherapy induced nausea and vomiting in children. Clin Oncol 5 : 11–14

19. Hirota T, Honjo T, Kuroda R, Saeki K, Katano N, Sakakibara Y, Shimizu H, Fujimoto T (1993) Antiemetic efficacy of granisetron in paediatric cancer treatment. Comparison of granisetron and granisetron plus methylprednisolone as antiemetic prophylaxis. Gan To Kagaku Ryoho 20 : 2369–2373

20. Holdsworth MT, Raisch DW, Duncan MH, Chavez CM, Leasure MM (1995) Assessment of chemotherapy-induced emesis and evaluation of a reduced-dose intravenous ondansetron regimen in paediatric outpatients with leukaemia. Ann Pharmacother 29 : 16–21

21. Jacobson SJ, Shore RW, Greenberg M, Spielberg SP (1994) The efficacy and safety of granisetron in paediatric cancer patients who had failed standard antiemetic therapy during anticancer chemotherapy. Am J Pediatr Hematol Oncol 16 : 231–235

22. Jurgens H, McQuade B (1992) Ondansetron as prophylaxis for chemotherapy and radiotherapy-induced emesis in children. Oncology 49 : 279–285

23. LeBaron S, Zeltzer LK, LeBaron C, Scott SE, Zeltzer PM (1988) Chemotherapy side effects in paediatric oncology patients: drugs, age, and sex as risk factors. Med Pediatr Oncol 16 : 269–270

24. Leclerc JM, Jacobson SJ, Cohn R, Pinkerton CR, Mee D, Nishimura L, Cedar E (1993) A double-blind dose-ranging study of i.v. granisetron in children undergoing highly emetogenic chemotherapy. Proc Am Soc Clin Oncol 12 : 437

25. Leclerc JM, Greenberg M, Lau R, Ingram L, Grant R, Howard D, Lariviere L, Perrotta M, Dempsey E (1995) Open label i.v. dolasetron mesylate in paediatric patients receiving moderately to highly emetogenic chemotherapy: pharmacokinetics, efficacy and safety. Support Care Cancer 3 : 343

26. Lemerle J, Amaral D, Southall DP, Upward J, Murdoch RD (1991) Efficacy and safety of granisetron in the prevention of chemotherapy-induced emesis in paediatric patients. Eur J Cancer 27 : 1081–1083

27. Marshall G, Kerr S, Vowels M, O'Gorman-Hughes D, White L (1989) Antiemetic therapy for chemotherapy-induced vomiting: metoclopramide, benztropine, dexamethasone, and lorazepam regimen compared with chlorpromazine alone. J Pediatr 115 : 156–160

28. Metha P, Gross S, Graham-Pole J, Gardner R (1986) Methylprednisolone for chemotherapy induced emesis: a double-blind randomized trial in children. J Pediatr 108 : 774–776

29. Miyajima Y, Numata S, Katayama I, Horibe K (1994) Prevention of chemotherapy-induced emesis with granisetron in children with malignant diseases. Am J Pediatr Hematol Oncol 16 : 236–241

30. Ninane J, Ozkaynak F, Kurtin P, Siegel SE (1995) Variation in the use of ondansetron as an antiemetic drug in children treated with chemotherapy. Med Pediatr Oncol 25 : 33–37

31. Panzarella C, Sallan SE, Carron GJ, House KW (1994) Intravenous plus oral ondansetron for prevention of emesis in children receiving chemotherapy. Proc Am Soc Clin Oncol 13 : 468

32. Patel N, Hunt J, McElwain T (1983) A comparison of the antiemetic efficacy and safety of nabilone and prochlorperazine in paediatric patients with cytotoxic-induced nausea and vomiting. Proceedings of the Second European Conference on Clinical Oncology, Amsterdam, 1983, 299

33. Rosso P, Cordero di Montezemolo L, Vivenza C, Nasi C, Tonello M, Valle P, Madon E (1994) Efficacy of tropisetron (Navoban®) in controlling emesis induced in children by anti-cancer therapy. Tumori 80 : 459–463

34. Suarez A, Stettler ER, Rey E, Pons G, Simonetta-Chateauneuf C, de Bruijn KM, Olive G, Lemerle J (1994) Safety, tolerability, efficacy and plasma concentrations of tropisetron after administration at five dose levels to children receiving cancer chemotherapy. Eur J Cancer 30A : 1436–1441
35. Sullivan MJ, Abbott GD, Robinson BA (1992) Ondansetron antiemetic therapy for chemotherapy and radiotherapy induced vomiting in children. NZ Med J 105 : 369–371
36. Swann IL, Thompson EN, Qureshi K (1979) Domperidone or metoclopramide in preventing chemotherapeutically induced nausea and vomiting. Br Med J 2 : 1979
37. Terrin BN, McWilliams NB, Maurer HM (1984) Side effects of metoclopramide as an antiemetic in childhood cancer chemotherapy. J Pediatr 104 : 138–140
38. Yanofsky R, Pyesmany A, Pritchard S, Leclerc SM, Pratt CB, Baker D, Howard D, Lariviere L, Perrotta M, Dempsey E (1995) Open label oral dolasetron mesylate in paediatric patients receiving moderately to highly emetogenic chemotherapy: pharmacokinetics, efficacy and safety. Support Care Cancer 3 : 344
39. Zeltzer L, LeBaron S, Zeltzer PM (1984) Paradoxical effects of prophylactic phenothiazine antiemetics in children receiving chemotherapy. J Clin Oncol 2 : 930–936

Methodology of Antiemetic Trials: Response Assessment, Evaluation of New Agents, and Definition of Chemotherapy Emetogenicity

Paul J. Hesketh, Richard J. Gralla, Andreas du Bois, Maurizio Tonato

ABSTRACT Establishing appropriate and practical methodology is a key to progress in the investigation of chemotherapy-induced nausea and vomiting. Critical issues include patient response assessment, proper trial design for evaluating new agents, and the definition of chemotherapy emetogenicity. In assessing antiemetic response, the primary end-point should be complete control of emesis and nausea. Emesis and nausea should be independently assessed with the period of observation defined (acute, delayed, anticipatory). Emesis can be evaluated by measuring the number of emetic episodes either by direct observation or by patient self-report using patient-completed diaries. Nausea should be measured by patient self-report with the standard parameters, including frequency and intensity. New antiemetic drug development should proceed in an orderly progression from open-label phase I/II trials defining tolerance and minimally fully effective dose to phase III comparative trials. A randomized, parallel, double-blind study is the preferred design for the latter, and the comparator arm should always include the current best available treatment. Antiemetic placebos are no longer acceptable with chemotherapy regimens known to produce emesis in a majority of patients. None of the emetogenic classifications proposed to date adequately accounts for all known important patient- and treatment-related prognostic variables. A modification of a recently reported schema is proposed for use in making antiemetic treatment recommendations and defining the emetogenic challenge in clinical trials.

Introduction

Significant progress has been made over the past 15 years in the development of more effective and better tolerated means of preventing chemotherapy-induced nausea and vomiting in cancer patients [15]. Control of emesis remains less than optimal, however, in a number of situations, including delayed emesis following cisplatin and emesis induced by very high dose chemotherapy. Therefore, there is a need to evaluate additional novel treatment approaches and new agents.

Establishing and employing practical methodology is a key to progress in the investigation of emesis and its control. Progress in the past was impeded by lack of a focus on the major end points and by varying methodology of questionable psychometric properties. Appropriate trial design improves the efficiency of new treatment evaluation, maximizes the interpretability of trial results, and allows for meaningful comparison of results across studies. Sound methodology also minimizes the chance that patients participating in antiemetic trials will be placed at unacceptable risk for emesis or excessive toxicity.

A number of reviews have previously addressed the issue of antiemetic trial methodology [1, 14, 28, 31, 32]. Although there is reasonable consistency among the latter on many issues, variation among antiemetic trials with respect to key methodologic issues continues to be seen. This manuscript will review a number of areas relating to antiemetic trial methodology, including patient response assessment, evaluation of new agents, and definition of chemotherapy emetogenicity. Consensus recommendations of the Fifth Perugia International Cancer Conference pertaining to these latter areas will be presented.

Assessment of Patient Response

Methods of data collection

Vomiting and retching (nonproductive vomiting), collectively termed emesis, can be objectively quantitated by measuring the number of emetic episodes (Table 1). Direct observation of the patient is an accurate and reliable technique to quantitate emetic episodes [13]. For patients treated in settings where prolonged direct observation is not possible, daily diary cards completed by patients have also proven reliable [12, 29] and are preferable to follow-up by telephone or questioning at the next clinic visit [29].

In delayed emesis trials, the use of questionnaires completed by the patient at home each day during the period of interest (usually 4–7 days) has been an effective method with high patient acceptance. Yield is increased by daily telephone contact.

The recording of emetic episodes when vomiting and retching occur almost continuously has been a vexing problem, with innumerable definitions used to characterize discrete emetic episodes [17, 21, 22]. One definition that simplifies this process considers a discrete emetic episode (vomiting and/or retching) to have ended when at least 1 min has passed since retching or vomiting ceased [21].

Table 1 Consensus recommendations on assessment of patient response (*EE* emetic episodes)

Recommendation	Level of consensus	Confidence level
Methods of data collection (see text for details)	High	High
Periods of assessment		
Acute: 24 h after chemotherapy	High	Moderate to high
Delayed: >24 h after chemotherapy	High	Moderate
Composite: 1–3 days after chemotherapy	Moderate to high	Moderate
End Points		
Primary		
Complete prevention of emesis		
(Complete response 0 EE)	High	High
Complete prevention of nausea	High	High
Secondary		
Major response	Moderate to high	Moderate
(0–2 EE)		
Other	Low	Low
(See text for details)		

Other parameters that have been measured with respect to emesis include volume of emesis, duration of emesis (either from the time of chemotherapy administration or from the initial episode to the cessation of emesis), and the time of onset of the first emetic episode.

The assessment of nausea has been a more challenging problem than that of emesis, given its subjective nature. Despite the good correlation between vomiting and nausea, they are distinct entities and should be separately evaluated. Although observer-rated reports of nausea have occasionally been employed [20, 26], the preferred method of assessment is patient self-report. The three primary characteristics of nausea that have been most commonly measured are frequency, intensity, and duration. Frequency is easily determined by patients providing a simple yes/no answer to specific questioning or through the use of a multipoint scale. Intensity of nausea has been assessed most commonly by means of visual analogue or descriptive ordinal scales [3, 11, 27]. Two studies simultaneously assessing nausea with different scales found a high correlation between a four-point descriptive scale (none, mild, moderate, severe) and visual analogue scales [8, 16]. One of these studies also evaluated the sensitivity of these scales and found them to be comparable [8].

Duration of nausea has been reported much less commonly in antiemetic trials than frequency and intensity [9]. Potential problems with this parameter include the need to rely on patient recall, which can be affected both by the frequency of assessments and concurrent medications and events. In addition, there is no commonly accepted method of measuring nausea duration.

Delfavero et al. have described two additional means of measuring nausea that provide composite measurements. These include entity and quantity of nausea [8]. To employ these composite measurements, assessments of nausea are carried out at a number of intervals during the study period. Entity is defined as the sum of all values of intensity of nausea recorded at each evaluation time point. Quantity is defined as the sum of the products of the intensity multiplied by the duration recorded at each evaluation time point. The potential advantage of the composite measurements is their greater sensitivity compared with unidimensional parameters. Therefore, they may provide a means to detect subtle clinical differences in comparative trials. Their major disadvantages, which argue against their general acceptance at present, are their added complexity and the limited experience with these measurements to date.

Period of Assessment

Periods of assessment for various emetic problems have been defined empirically (Table 1). Acute chemotherapy-induced emesis is the most common problem. It has been defined as that emesis occurring in the first 24 h after the administration of chemotherapy. The 24-h period serves to separate evaluation of the problem from that of delayed emesis. This definition is useful in delineating the two problems, but is not necessarily based on an identified physiological or neuropharmacological difference. It is also useful in that most emesis occurs during this period if effective treatment is not given. Assessment also includes the evaluation of nausea during the period of the emetic problem.

Late-onset emesis is a subtype of acute emesis that has been defined for agents such as cyclophosphamide and carboplatin, which tend to induce emesis much later than most chemotherapy agents, typically at 12 h or more after chemotherapy [11, 25].

Delayed emesis is differentiated from acute or late-onset emesis by an arbitrary definition. It is defined as that emesis starting (or persisting) after the initial 24-h period. This definition has served us well in the identification of the problem and been helpful in the study of control of delayed emesis. There are several theories on the neuropharmacology of the problem; however, these hypotheses remain controversial. The exact time of onset of delayed emesis is not clear, but it has been suggested that it may commonly begin a few hours earlier than the definition. The period of assessment for delayed emesis has varied with different chemotherapy regimens. Following cisplatin, the period of assessment has most commonly extended from the second to the fifth day after chemotherapy. With other chemotherapy regimens, assessment periods have most commonly extended from 3 to 5 days after chemotherapy. As long as the pathophysiology of both acute and delayed emesis remains unclear, cutoffs between these two entities will always be arbitrary and recommendations for clinical studies will remain vague. One way to overcome these limitations is to focus on total control of emesis over a chemotherapy course as a whole. For practical reasons, the observation period might be limited to 3 days following chemotherapy administration, because almost all patients who vomit will start vomiting within the first 3 days.

Anticipatory or conditioned emesis is often defined as that emesis beginning prior to the administration of chemotherapy in patients who have previously received chemotherapy. It is clear that poor control of acute or delayed emesis predisposes to this problem.

Response Criteria

Primary End Points

The gold standard for antiemetic response is the complete prevention of all emesis and nausea. Emesis is best quantitated by assessing the number of emetic (vomiting/retching) episodes. The primary end-point for emesis is complete response, defined as no emetic episodes during the specified observation period (Table 1).

Given its subjective and distinctive nature, nausea should be assessed independently of emesis. Notably, control of nausea has consistently been inferior to control of emesis in clinical trials, with complete nausea control rates approximately 10% lower than complete control rates for emesis [8]. The primary efficacy end points should be the frequency and intensity of nausea. The latter can be determined equally well with descriptive ordinal or visual analogue scales.

A new category of total control has recently emerged and is defined as the complete control of both emesis and nausea. It is unclear whether this new category adds substantially to existing response criteria, as total control rates in most reports are typically very similar to the complete control rates are of nausea.

Secondary End Points

A number of additional response categories have been defined by the number of emetic episodes. These include: major (≤ 2 emetic episodes), minor (3–5 emetic episodes), and failure (>5 emetic episodes). The major response category continues to be useful in assessing antiemetic treatment benefit and should be retained as a secondary end point for response. The clinical utility of the traditional minor and failure categories has become increasingly suspect as antiemetic treatment for conventional-dose chemotherapy has improved. A new failure category, defined as more than two emetic episodes, should be considered. In addition, use of rescue antiemetics and withdrawal from the study should also be classed as failure. After the use of rescue antiemetics, patient observation should continue for the full study period nonetheless, with a complete recording of the total number of emetic episodes.

The complete and major control categories have been helpful in assessing delayed emesis in addition to acute emesis. In delayed emesis, it can be useful to report the number of episodes by each of the first 4 or 5 days after chemotherapy and control over the entire delayed emesis risk period. In assessing anticipatory nausea or vomiting, it is sufficient simply to report on the presence or absence of the problem.

Other End Points

Other parameters that have been measured with respect to emesis include volume and duration of emesis. However, neither can be recommended for primary or secondary end points. Volume of emesis is difficult to measure, is dependent on oral intake, and is not clinically useful [31]. Duration of emesis has been recorded by a number of groups, but no standard definition has yet emerged to characterize this parameter. Time to first emetic episode (mean or median) has also been employed in assessing response. Although not a primary end-point, it may occasionally have value in comparative antiemetic trials.

Other parameters that have been employed in assessing nausea include duration, time to nausea, and composite measurements, such as entity and quantity. None should be considered as primary or secondary end points at the present time.

Evaluating New Agents

New antiemetic drug development should follow an orderly and logical progression beginning with open-label phase I/II tolerance and dose-finding trials and progressing through phase III comparative trials (Table 2). Appropriate candidates for phase I trials are normal volunteers or cancer patients who have failed prior conventional antiemetic treatments. In this type of trial, efficacy parameters are important, but clearly secondary to toxicity assessments. After successful completion of phase I trials, phase II trials should be completed to confirm antiemetic efficacy and define minimally fully effec-

Table 2 Consensus recommendations on evaluation of new agents

Recommendation	Level of consensus	Confidence level
1. Phase I/II trials should always precede phase III trials	High	High
2. Phase I/II trials should define minimal fully effective dose	High	High
3. Phase III trials should employ a double-blind, randomized parallel design	High	High
4. Phase III trials should use best available treatment as comparators	High	High
5. Placebo comparators are not appropriate for trials of acute emesis with moderately or highly emetogenic chemotherapy or trials of delayed emesis after high-dose cisplatin (see text)	High	High

tive doses. Appropriate study populations for phase II trials are patients failing conventional treatment. If substantial efficacy is noted in initial studies, then appropriate additional populations for study include chemotherapy-naive patients receiving moderately to highly emetogenic chemotherapy.

Phase III trials should be initiated only after completion of phase I/II trials. A prerandomization stratification for important prognostic variables such as gender and ethanol consumption should be required unless a large sample population of patients is enrolled in the study and the impact of prognostic factors is analyzed by a multifactorial analysis at the end of the study. A randomized, parallel double-blind study is the preferred design for comparative trials. The comparator arm should always contain the current best available treatment. If efficacy results of phase II trials are sufficiently compelling, then the new agent can be compared as a single agent against the best available therapy. An acceptable alternative design is to combine the new agent with the current best standard and compare it with the current best standard combined with placebo.

Treatment with antiemetic placebos alone is no longer acceptable with chemotherapies known to induce emesis in most patients. This includes the evaluation of acute emesis with moderately to highly emetogenic chemotherapy and delayed emesis in patients receiving high-dose cisplatin (100 mg/m^2). Use of placebos in delayed emesis following lower-dose cisplatin and non-cisplatin-based chemotherapy remains controversial and should be further evaluated. In either of the latter instances, if a placebo treatment is employed, there should be zero tolerance for the development of any breakthrough emesis or nausea, with immediate rescue of patients developing symptoms.

A key element in new agent and new regimen evaluation is a careful assessment of the side effect profile. This includes objectively measurable side effects, such as changes in vital signs, blood chemistries, electrocardiograms, or physical examinations, which are typically scored using the NCI common criteria. In addition, subjectively measurable side effects, such as headache, akathisia, sedation, and diarrhea, should also be assessed. Typically these effects are measured by their presence or absence and then with a categorical rating by the patient (mild, moderate, or severe effects). An ongoing challenge in the evaluation of the side effects of new agents is separating the adverse effects of the antiemetics from those of the chemotherapy, symptoms of the malignancy, intercurrent illnesses, or concomitant medications.

Defining Chemotherapy Emetogenicity

Defining the emetogenicity of chemotherapy agents is of value for at least two important reasons. Such a classification can be used as a framework for defining antiemetic treatment guidelines. Secondly, it can provide a means for clinical investigators to attain a more precise definition of the emetogenic challenge that is being employed in an antiemetic trial. A useful schema would provide enough information to be utilized for both of these purposes. At present there is no commonly accepted schema for classifying the emetogenicity of cancer chemotherapy agents or combinations. A number of schemas have been proposed in which chemotherapy agents have been divided among three to five emetogenic levels [1, 4, 23, 24, 30]. The literature has been a very limited source of useful information in the development of these schemas, given the imprecise, inconsistent, and extremely limited ways in which information on emesis and nausea has been recorded in most therapeutic trials. Most schemas have not differentiated between the various types of emesis, such as acute, delayed, and anticipatory, and few have accounted for important treatment- and patient-related variables, such as chemotherapy dose, rate and route of administration, gender, age, and history of ethanol consumption [7, 18].

Recently Hesketh et al. proposed a classification system for acute emesis that accounts for chemotherapy dose and standardizes the rate and route of chemotherapy administration [19]. Chemotherapy agents were divided into five levels according to the expected frequency of emesis in the absence of effective antiemetic prophylaxis. Given the paucity of objective data in the literature, however, this schema, like others proposed earlier, reflects primarily

Table 3 Consensus recommendations on defining emetogenicity of chemotherapy

Recommendations	Level of consensus	Confidence level
1. Emetic potential and pattern of emesis should be rigorously assessed during clinical development of new agents	High	High
2. Comprehensive schema for classifying chemotherapy emetogenicity incorporating all important treatment and patient-related prognostic variables not currently available	High	High
3. Descriptive classification based upon clinical database of homogeneously treated patients should be established	High	Moderate
4. Working schema for use in defining emetogenicity for antiemetic trials and for development of treatment guidelines proposed (see Table 4)	Moderate	Low

the opinions of the authors and is thus potentially open to some of the criticisms that have been directed at prior schemas.

Hesketh et al. also proposed an algorithm to define the acute emetogenicity of chemotherapy combinations [19]. It was partially validated by analyzing a database of patients treated with placebos on clinical trials with ondansetron [2, 5, 6, 10]. The primary limitation of this algorithm is the relatively homogeneous nature of the patient sample on which it was validated (primarily women with breast cancer receiving cyclophosphamide-based chemotherapy). Its potential applicability in more heterogeneous populations receiving non-cyclophosphamide-based regimens remains to be determined.

At present, no single schema addresses all of the important issues that must be taken into account in defining a definitive emetogenic classification system, and further work should be carried out on this important issue (Table 3). One potential area in which new information can be obtained relates to the emetogenic potential of new cytotoxic agents. During the initial evaluation process of a new cytotoxic agent, there is a unique opportunity to obtain definitive information on the emetogenic potential and pattern of emesis in the absence of routine antiemetic treatment. Such information should be routinely recorded during new drug development.

Another potential approach to defining chemotherapy emetogenicity would be to analyze large databases in which information on emesis has been prospectively recorded and antiemetic prophylaxis was uniform. Such an

Table 4 Approximate emetogenic potential of single chemotherapy agents

Degree of emetogenicity	Agents
High	Cisplatin ≥ 50 mg/m^2 Mechlorethamine Streptozocin Cyclophosphamide >1500 mg/m^2 Carmustine >250 mg/m^2 Dacarbazine
Moderate to high	Cisplatin <50 mg/m^2 Cytarabine >1 gm/m^2 Carboplatin Ifosfamide Carmustine ≤ 250 mg/m^2 Hexamethylmelamine (p.o.) Cyclophosphamide ≤ 1500 mg/m^2 Anthracyclines Topotecan Irinotecan Procarbazine (p.o.) Methotrexate >250 mg/m^2 Cyclophosphamide (p.o.) Mitoxantrone
Low to moderate	Taxoids Etoposide Methotrexate >50 mg/m$^2 <250$ mg/m^2 Mitomycin Gemcitabine Fluorouracil <1000 mg/m^2
Low	Bleomycin Busulfan Chlorambucil (p.o.) 2-Chlorodeoxyadenosine Fludarabine Hydroxyurea Methotrexate ≤ 50 mg/m^2 L-phenylalanine mustard (p.o.) 6-Thioguanine (p.o.) Vinblastine Vincristine Vinorelbine

analysis could provide information on relative emetogenicity and potentially permit gender and other important prognostic variables to be accounted for as well.

Despite the limitations of all the emetogenic classification schemas proposed to date, there is still a need to agree upon a working schema than can be employed for treatment recommendations and for defining the emetogenic challenge in clinical trials. For this purpose, a modification of the schema of Hesketh et al. is proposed (Table 4). Chemotherapy agents are listed in order of decreasing emetogenicity with division across four broad emetogenic groups: high, moderate–high, low–moderate, and low.

References

1. Aapro M (1993) Methodological issues in antiemetic studies. Investigational New Drugs 11 : 243–253
2. Beck TM, Ciociola AA, Jones SE et al (1993) Efficacy of oral ondansetron in the prevention of emesis in outpatients receiving cyclophosphamide-based chemotherapy. Ann Intern Med 118 : 407–413
3. Clark RA, Tyson LB, Frisone M (1985) A correlation of objective and subjective parameters in assessing anti-emetic regimens. Proc Tenth Ann Cong Oncol Nurs Soc 2 : 96
4. Craig JB, Powell BL (1987) The management of nausea and vomiting in clinical oncology (review). Am J Med Sci 34–44
5. Cubeddu LX, Hoffman IS, Fuenmayor NT et al (1990) Antagonism of serotonin S3 receptors with ondansetron prevents nausea and emesis induced by cyclophosphamide-containing chemotherapy regimens. J Clin Oncol 8 : 1721–1727
6. Cubeddu LX, Pendergrass K, Ryan T et al (1994) Efficacy of oral ondansetron, a selective antagonist of 5-HT$_3$ receptors, in the treatment of nausea and vomiting associated with cyclophosphamide-based chemotherapy. Am J Clin Oncol 17 : 137–146
7. D'Acquisto R, Tyson LB, Gralla RJ et al (1986) The influence of a chronic high alcohol intake on chemotherapy-induced nausea and vomiting. Proc Am Soc Clin Oncol 5 : 257
8. DelFavero A, Roila F, Basurto C et al (1990) Assessment of nausea. Eur J Clin Pharmacol 38 : 115
9. DelFavero A, Tonato M, Roila F (1992) Issues in the measurement of nausea. Br J Cancer 66 [Suppl] : S69–S71
10. DiBenedetto J Jr, Cubeddu LX, Ryan T et al (1995) Ondansetron for nausea and vomiting associated with moderately emetogenic cancer chemotherapy. Clin Ther 17 : 1091–1098
11. Fetting JH, Grochow LB, Folstein MF et al (1982) The course of nausea and vomiting after high-dose cyclophosphamide. Cancer Treat Rep 66 : 1487–1493
12. Geddes DM, Dones L, Hill E et al (1990) Quality of life during chemotherapy for small cell lung cancer: assessment and use of a daily diary card in a randomized trial. Eur J Cancer 26 : 484–492
13. Gralla RJ, Itri LM, Pisko SE et al (1981) Antiemetic efficacy of high-dose metoclopramide: randomized trials with placebo and prochlorperazine in patients with chemotherapy-induced nausea and vomiting. N Engl J Med 305 : 905–909
14. Gralla RJ, Clark RA, Kris MG et al (1991) Methodology in anti-emetic trials. Eur J Cancer 27 : S5–S8

15. Grunberg SM, Hesketh PJ (1993) Control of chemotherapy-induced emesis. N Engl J Med 329 : 1790–1796

16. Havsteen H, Nielsen H, Kiaer M (1986) The use of visual analogue scale (VAS) in patients receiving cisplatin-containing chemotherapy. Proc Am Soc Clin Oncol 5 : 263

17. Hesketh PJ, Murphy WK, Lester EP et al (1989) GR 38032F (GR-C507/75): a novel compound effective in the prevention of acute cisplatin-induced emesis. J Clin Oncol 7 : 700–705

18. Hesketh PJ, Plagge P, Bryson JC (1992) Single-dose ondansetron for prevention of acute cisplatin-induced emesis: analysis of efficacy and prognostic factors. In: Bianchi AL, Grelot L, Miller AD, King GL (eds) Mechanisms and control of emesis. John Libbey, London, pp 25–26

19. Hesketh PJ, Kris MG, Grunberg SM et al (1997) Proposal for classifying the acute emetogenicity of cancer chemotherapy. J Clin Oncol 15 : 103–109

20. Holmes S, Eburn E (1989) Patients' and nurses' perceptions of symptom distress in cancer. J Adv Nurs 14 : 840–846

21. Italian Group for Antiemetic Research (1995) Dexamethasone, granisetron, or both for the prevention of nausea and vomiting during chemotherapy for cancer. N Engl J Med 332 : 1–5

22. Kris MG, Gralla RJ, Clark RA et al (1985) Consecutive dose-finding trials adding lorazepam to the combination of metoclopramide plus dexamethasone: improved subjective effectiveness over the combination of diphenhydramine plus metoclopramide plus dexamethasone. Cancer Treat Rep 69 : 1257–1262

23. Laszlo J (1982) Treatment of nausea and vomiting caused by cancer chemotherapy. Cancer Treat Rev 9 : 3–9

24. Lindley CM, Bernard S, Fields SM (1989) Incidence and duration of chemotherapy-induced nausea and vomiting in the outpatient oncology population. J Clin Oncol 7 : 1142–1149

25. Martin M, Diaz Rubio E, Sanchez A et al (1990) The natural course of emesis after carboplatin treatment. Acta Oncologica 29 : 593–596

26. Melzack R (1989) Measurement of nausea. J Pain Symptom Manage 4 : 157–160

27. Morrow GR (1984) The assessment of nausea and vomiting: past problems, current issues, and suggestions for future research. Cancer 53 [Suppl] : 2267–2278

28. Olver IN, Simon RM, Aisner J (1986) Antiemetic studies: a methodological discussion. Cancer Treat Rep 70 : 555–563

29. Smyth JF (1988) The problem of emesis induced by cancer chemotherapy. Clinician 6 : 2–12

30. Strum SB, McDermed JE, Pileggi J et al (1984) Intravenous metoclopramide: prevention of chemotherapy-induced nausea and vomiting. Cancer 53 : 1432–1439

31. Tonato M, Roila F, DelFavero A (1991) Methodology of antiemetic trials: a review. Ann Oncol 2 : 107–114

32. Tonato M, Roila F, DelFavero A (1996) Methodology of trials with antiemetics. Support Care Cancer 4 : 281–286

Delayed Emesis Following Anticancer Chemotherapy

Mark G. Kris, Fausto Roila, Pieter H.M. De Mulder, Michel Marty

ABSTRACT Delayed emesis is a distinct syndrome where vomiting begins or persists 24 or more hours after chemotherapy. It is more likely to occur when the stimulus for emesis is strong and/or acute vomiting is poorly controlled. The pathophysiology appears different than that which causes acute emesis. The literature reporting clinical trials to prevent delayed nausea and vomiting is presented. The best ways of preventing delayed emesis following anticancer chemotherapy are discussed.

Introduction

Once vomiting was prevented on the day of chemotherapy in the majority of patients, it became apparent that many individuals experienced delayed emesis 1 or more days afterward. This syndrome was first described in patients receiving cisplatin given at doses of 120 mg/m^2; 74% developed delayed vomiting and 87% delayed nausea during the period from 24 h to 120 h after chemotherapy [13].

Delayed symptoms also occur with lower doses of cisplatin [32], cyclophosphamide [2, 12], doxorubicin and epirubicin [11], and carboplatin [11, 30].

Definition

Delayed emesis was initially defined as vomiting occurring 24 h or more after chemotherapy and included any vomiting episodes occurring 24–144 h after cisplatin [13].

Individuals with no acute vomiting were found to be less likely to experience delayed vomiting. The incidence of delayed vomiting following cisplatin is greatest for the 24-h period from 48 to 72 h after cisplatin and from 24 to 48 h after cyclophosphamide and progressively declines in the successive 24-h periods for both chemotherapy drugs. Because of the low incidence of vomiting seen on the later days, several authors have shortened the treatment and observation period for delayed emesis to 120 [16] or 96 h [28]. The period from 24 h to 96 h after chemotherapy includes the time of greatest incidence and requirement for prophylaxis or rescue treatment. This 3-day interval is the minimal time period that should be studied in trials addressing this syndrome and for which preventative treatment for this condition should be given.

When does delayed emesis begin? The current 24-h cutoff was empirically chosen to define an easily obtainable starting point for clinical studies. When the time-course of emesis is plotted for the period from 0 to 24 h after cisplatin in patients given placebo antiemetics or metoclopramide, a biphasic pattern is observed, with an initial period of intense emesis from 2 to 12 h and a "second peak" beginning approximately 18 h after chemotherapy [18, 19]. Even in patients given placebo antiemetics with cisplatin, emesis ceases temporarily between the two phases. Ondansetron given as a single agent, so effective during the first 12 h, was much less so from 16 h to 24 h, when the majority of "failures" occurred [14, 15]. Recently it has been postulated that the "second peak", beginning about 16 h after cisplatin, is actually the true onset of delayed emesis [18]. In contrast, among patients who fail prophylaxis with a 5-HT$_3$ antagonist plus dexamethasone, vomiting can start at any time during the first 24 h, without clear peaks and without interruption [27]. One early trial has shown improved control of delayed emesis when prophylactic antiemetics are started 16 h after cisplatin [29]. From a practical standpoint, it appears reasonable to measure and initiate therapy for delayed emesis the morning after chemotherapy is administered, which generally works out to be 16–24 h afterward.

Pathophysiology

As in the case of chemotherapy-induced emesis in general, we have not yet elucidated the exact mechanisms that underlie delayed emesis. Several authors have postulated that the pathways and neurotransmitters mediating delayed emesis differ from those mediating acute emesis, since the pharmacological agents that are uniformly effective in the acute phase are much less so during the delayed period. No experimental model of delayed emesis is universally accepted. The ferrets used in the model of Florczyk et al. [5] are routinely sacrificed after only a 4-h observation period. When the animals are observed for longer periods, the pattern of acute and delayed emesis seen in man does not occur when the ferrets are given the 10 mg/kg routine cisplatin dose [34]. Recently, Rudd and Naylor have demonstrated an acute and delayed emesis pattern in ferrets given 5 mg/kg of cisplatin, which was very similar to that seen in patients [34]. Milano and colleagues have developed a piglet model of delayed emesis that appears to be granisetron responsive, an observation that does not accurately reflect the limited effectiveness of the 5-HT$_3$ antagonists when used to treat delayed emesis in man [22].

Whether either of these two models will become a standard remains in question. Recently, non-peptide substance P antagonists, which block the NK$_1$ receptor, have demonstrated the ability to lessen delayed emesis in animals [33]. In preliminary trials in man, single doses of the substance P antagonist CP-122,721 prevented delayed emesis in 83% of patients receiving over 100 mg/m^2 cisplatin, including individuals who had experienced delayed symptoms in earlier cisplatin cycles [20]. These observations suggest that the NK$_1$ receptor and its natural ligand substance P may play a part in the delayed emetic reflex.

Treatment of Delayed Emesis After Cisplatin

The vast majority of trials attempting to prevent delayed emesis have been conducted in patients receiving cisplatin (Table 1). No studies have addressed the treatment of ongoing delayed emesis. The first trials designed to prevent delayed emesis tested agents and combinations useful in the treatment of acute cisplatin-induced emesis, including metoclopramide alone [7, 32] and metoclopramide or prochlorperazine plus dexamethasone [1, 35]. In a randomized, placebo-controlled trial, dexamethasone prevented delayed emesis in 35% of patients receiving cisplatin 120 mg/m^2, and the combination of dexamethasone plus metoclopramide in 52% [16]. Subsequent trials have confirmed the effectiveness and safety of the metoclopramide plus corticosteroid combination [23, 28]. ACTH has also been shown to prevent delayed emesis in placebo-controlled trials among cisplatin-treated patients [25].

The initial trials of the specific serotonin antagonist ondansetron [3, 6, 8, 17, 21, 31] failed to demonstrate a degree of benefit equal to that seen with this agent when used to treat acute emesis. Many of these trials, however, were not specifically designed to test treatments for delayed emesis. Because the control of acute emesis varied, and it is well established that vomiting during the initial 24 h after chemotherapy is one of the strongest factors predicting delayed emesis, the usefulness of these data for the understanding and control of delayed vomiting is inherently limited. A large placebo-controlled trial demonstrated minimal activity of ondansetron in preventing delayed emesis, but the results are difficult to interpret because of reporting flaws [24]. A recent randomized study demonstrated equivalent delayed antiemetic prevention for metoclopramide and ondansetron when each was combined with dexamethasone [28]. Among patients who vomited in the first 24 h, however, ondansetron plus dexamethasone provided better complete protection from

Table 1 Regimens to prevent delayed emesis after cisplatin

Initiation	The morning following cisplatin	
Duration	Three to five days following chemotherapy (approximate time from 72 to 144 h)	
Regimens	Dexamethasone	8 mg p.o. twice daily for 2 days then 4 mg p.o. twice daily for 2 days
	Plus Metoclopramide 0.5 mg/kg p.o. four times daily for 4 days [16]	
	Dexamethasone	8 mg i.m. twice daily for 2 days then 4 mg i.m. twice daily for 1 day
	Plus either: Metoclopramide 20 mg p.o. every 6 h for 3 days or Ondansetron 8 mg p.o. every 12 h for 3 days [28]	

vomiting than the metoclopramide-containing regimen (29% versus 9%) [28]. In a large, multicenter trial, the combination of granisetron plus dexamethasone was equivalent to dexamethasone alone [9].

Clinical trials have established the effectiveness of dexamethasone and combinations of dexamethasone plus either metoclopramide or a specific 5-HT_3 antagonist. The combination of dexamethasone with either metoclopramide or a 5-HT_3 antagonist represents the treatment of choice to prevent delayed emesis after cisplatin.

Treatment of Delayed Emesis After Cyclophosphamide

Cyclophosphamide given at doses of 50–75 mg/kg has been shown to cause vomiting more than 24 h later [4].

In another trial among patients receiving 500–600 mg/m^2 cyclophosphamide and placebo antiemetics, 33% experienced emesis from 24 to 96 h after chemotherapy [2].

In addition to cyclophosphamide, delayed nausea and vomiting also follow other "moderately emetogenic chemotherapy," including that with such agents as doxorubicin (>40 mg/m^2 alone and >25 mg/m^2 in combination), epirubicin (>75 mg/m^2 alone or >50 mg/m^2 in combination), and carboplatin (>300 mg/m^2) (Table 2) [11].

Table 2 Regimens to prevent delayed emesis after cyclophosphamide, doxorubicin, epirubicin, or carboplatin

Initiation	The morning following cyclophosphamide, doxorubicin, epirubicin, or carboplatin
Duration	Three to 6 days following chemotherapy (approximate time from 72 to 168 h)
Regimens	Dexamethasone 4 mg p.o. twice daily for 4 days [12]
	Ondansetron 8 mg p.o. every 12 h for 4 days [11]
	Dexamethasone 8 mg p.o. once daily for 6 days [26]
	Dolasetron 200 mg p.o. once daily for 6 days plus dexamethasone 8 mg p.o. once daily for 6 days [26]
	Ondansetron 8 mg p.o. twice daily for 6 days plus dexamethasone 8 mg p.o. once daily for 6 days [26]

In a randomized trial in which patients were given placebo antiemetics for delayed emesis caused by moderately emetogenic chemotherapy, 58% had delayed vomiting [11]. In a second trial among individuals given 750 mg/m^2 cyclophosphamide and placebo antiemetics, 67% suffered delayed vomiting [12].

Among patients receiving cyclophosphamide, dexamethasone [12] and ondansetron [11] have been found to be superior to placebo in controlling delayed vomiting. Among patients receiving carboplatin, epirubicin, and doxorubicin, ondansetron [11] was superior to placebo in preventing delayed emesis. Dolasetron or ondansetron, each combined with dexamethasone, prevented delayed emesis in 47% of patients, as against 41% prevention with dexamethasone alone ($p=0.24$) in a North American trial in which 407 individuals receiving cyclophosphamide, carboplatin, doxorubicin, and epirubicin were studied [26]. As was the case with cisplatin, delayed emesis was prospectively assessed as a secondary end point in many other trials. Because the control of acute emesis varied, and we know that vomiting during the initial 24 h after chemotherapy is one of the strongest factors predicting delayed emesis, the usefulness of these data for understanding and control of delayed vomiting is inherently limited. In the follow-up phase of a trial evaluating acute emesis prevention with ondansetron and placebo in cyclophosphamide-treated patients, ondansetron was superior in the prevention of both acute and delayed emesis [2]. When ondansetron was compared with dexamethasone, however, significantly more of the patients receiving dexamethasone (87%) than of those taking ondansetron (72%) reported control of delayed nausea ($p=0.003$) [10]. Delayed emesis was seen in 33% receiving dexamethasone and 48% receiving ondansetron in the same trial ($p=0.0.2$) [10]. In a randomized trial comparing granisetron alone, dexamethasone alone and the combination of dexamethasone plus granisetron for the control of acute emesis and observation with rescue for the delayed emesis period, conducted among patients receiving moderately emetogenic chemotherapy, the overall incidence of delayed vomiting was only 21% [30]. The same authors also noted that delayed vomiting occurred in only 12% of individuals with no acute vomiting, but in 54% in patients who had experienced acute vomiting. This observation has led to the proposal that only those patients who experience acute vomiting should receive prophylaxis for delayed vomiting. A trial is planned to test this idea.

Based on the data available from the completed trials, dexamethasone alone, a 5-HT$_3$ antagonist alone, or dexamethasone in combination with a 5-HT$_3$ antagonist is the most effective regimen to control delayed nausea and emesis following moderately emetogenic chemotherapy.

Consensus Proposal on Delayed Emesis Following Anticancer Therapy

1. Delayed emesis is a distinct syndrome following cisplatin and moderately emetogenic chemotherapy (especially cyclophosphamide and carboplatin), defined as vomiting that starts or continues the day following chemotherapy.

   Level of scientific confidence: High
   Level of consensus: High

2. Delayed emesis has been traditionally defined as commencing 24 h or more after chemotherapy. However, observations of emesis patterns in patients not receiving antiemetic prophylaxis suggest that this syndrome can begin as early as 16 h after cisplatin or beyond 24 h with cyclophosphamide.

   Level of scientific confidence: Moderate
   Level of consensus: High

3. All patients receiving cisplatin at doses over 50 mg/m^2 should receive antiemetic prophylaxis for delayed emesis.

   Level of scientific confidence: High
   Level of consensus: High

4. The combination of dexamethasone and either metoclopramide or a specific 5-HT$_3$ antagonist beginning the morning after and continuing for a minimum of 3 days (72 h) is the most effective regimen to prevent delayed emesis caused by cisplatin.

Level of scientific confidence:	High
Level of consensus:	High

5. The occurrence of cisplatin-induced delayed emesis in many patients despite prophylactic treatment with dexamethasone, metoclopramide, and specific serotonin antagonists suggests that delayed symptoms are only partially mediated by neurotransmitters affected by these agents. Research to characterize the pathophysiology of this syndrome is needed.

Level of scientific confidence:	Not applicable
Level of consensus:	High

6. If delayed emesis induced by moderately emetogenic chemotherapy is expected in more than 30% of patients, prophylactic treatment should be administered.

Level of scientific confidence:	Low
Level of consensus:	High

7. If prophylaxis for delayed emesis following moderately emetogenic chemotherapy is indicated, dexamethasone alone, a 5-HT$_3$ antagonist alone, or the combination of dexamethasone and a 5-HT$_3$ antagonist, beginning the morning after and continuing for a minimum of 3 days (72 h), should be administered.

Level of scientific confidence:	Moderate
Level of consensus:	Moderate

References

1. Clark R, Kris M, Tyson L, Gralla R, O'Hehir M (1986) Antiemetic trials to control delayed vomiting following high-dose cisplatin. Proc Am Soc Clin Oncol 5 : 257
2. Cubeddu LX, Hoffman IS, Fuenmayor NT, Finn AL (1990) Antagonism of serotonin S3 receptors with ondansetron prevents nausea and emesis induced by cyclophosphamide-containing chemotherapy regimens. J Clin Oncol 8 : 1721–1727
3. De Mulder PHM, Seynaeve C, Vermorken JB, van Liessum PA, Mols-Jevdevic S, Allman EL, Beranek P, Verweij J (1990) Ondansetron compared with high-dose metoclopramide in prophylaxis of acute and delayed cisplatin-induced nausea and vomiting. Ann Intern Med 113 : 834–840
4. Fetting JH, Grochow LB, Folstein MF, Ettinger DS, Colvin M (1982) The course of nausea and vomiting after high-dose cyclophosphamide. Cancer Treat Rep 66 : 1487–1493
5. Florczyk AP, Schurig JE, Bradner WT (1982) Cisplatin-induced emesis in the ferret: a new animal model. Cancer Treat Rep 66 : 187–189

6. Gandara DR, Harvey WH, Monaghan GG, Perez EA, Stokes C, Bryson JC, Finn AL, Hesketh PJ (1992) The delayed-emesis syndrome from cisplatin: phase III evaluation of ondansetron versus placebo. Semin Oncol 19 : 67–71

7. Grunberg SM, Ehler E, McDermed JE, Akerley WL (1988) Oral metoclopramide with or without diphenhydramine: potential for prevention of late nausea and vomiting induced by cisplatin. J Natl Cancer Inst 80 : 864–868

8. Grunberg SM, Groshen S, Stevenson LL, McDermed J, Lucci L, Sanderson PE (1990) Double blind randomized study of 2 doses of oral ondansetron (GR 38032F) for the prevention of cisplatin (C)-induced delayed nausea (N) and vomiting (V). Proc Am Soc Clin Oncol 9 : 327

9. Johnston D, Latreille J, Laberge F, Stewart D, Rusthoven J, Findlay B, Ernst S (1995) Preventing nausea and vomiting during days 2–7 following high dose cisplatin chemotherapy (HDCP). A study by the National Cancer Institute of Canada Clinical Trials Group (NCIC CTG). Proc Am Soc Clin Oncol 14 : 529

10. Jones AL, Hill AS, Soukop M, Hutcheon AW, Cassidy J, Kaye SB, Sikora K, Carney DN, Cunningham D (1991) Comparison of dexamethasone and ondansetron in the prophylaxis of emesis induced by moderately emetogenic chemotherapy. Lancet 338 : 483–487

11. Kaizer L, Warr D, Hoskins P, Latreille J, Lofters W, Yau J, Palmer M, Zee B, Levy M, Pater J (1994) Effect of schedule and maintenance on the antiemetic efficacy of ondansetron combined with dexamethasone in acute and delayed nausea and emesis in patients receiving moderately emetogenic chemotherapy: a phase III trial by the national cancer institute of Canada clinical trials group. J Clin Oncol 12 : 1050–1057

12. Koo WH, Ang PT (1996) Role of maintenance oral dexamethasone in prophylaxis of delayed emesis caused by moderately emetogenic chemotherapy. Ann Oncol 7 : 71–74

13. Kris MG, Gralla RJ, Clark RA, Tyson LB, OConnell JP, Wertheim MS, Kelsen DP (1985) Incidence, course, and severity of delayed nausea and vomiting following the administration of high-dose cisplatin. J Clin Oncol 3 : 1379–1384

14. Kris MG, Gralla RJ, Clark RA, Tyson LB (1988) Dose-ranging evaluation of the serotonin antagonist GR-C507/75 (GR38032F) when used as an antiemetic in patients receiving anticancer chemotherapy. J Clin Oncol 6 : 659–662

15. Kris MG, Gralla RJ, Clark RA, Tyson LB (1989) Phase II trials of the serotonin antagonist GR38032F for the control of vomiting caused by cisplatin. J Natl Cancer Inst 81 : 42–46

16. Kris MG, Gralla RJ, Tyson LB, Clark RA, Cirrincione C, Groshen S (1989) Controlling delayed vomiting: double-blind, randomized trial comparing placebo, dexamethasone alone, and metoclopramide plus dexamethasone in patients receiving cisplatin. J Clin Oncol 7 : 108–114

17. Kris MG, Tyson LB, Clark RA, Gralla RG (1992) Oral ondansetron for the control of delayed emesis after cisplatin. Report of a phase II study and a review of completed trials to manage delayed emesis. Cancer 70 : 1012–1016

18. Kris MG, Pisters KMW, Hinkley L (1994) Delayed emesis following anticancer chemotherapy. Support Care Cancer 2 : 297–300

19. Kris MG, Cubeddu LX, Gralla RJ, Cupissol D, Tyson LB, Venkatraman E, Homesley HD (1996) Are more antiemetic trials with placebo necessary? Report of patient data from randomized trials of placebo antiemetics with cisplatin. Cancer 78 : 2193–2198

20. Kris MG, Radford JE, Pizzo BA, Inabinet R, Hesketh A, Hesketh PJ (1997) Use of a NK-1 receptor antagonist to prevent delayed emesis following cisplatin. J Natl Cancer Inst 89 : 53–54

21. Marty M, Pouillart P, Scholl S, Droz JP, Azab M, Brion N, Pujade LE, Paule B, Paes D, Bons J (1990) Comparison of the 5-hydroxytryptamine 3 (serotonin) antagonist ondansetron (GR 38032F) with high-dose metoclopramide in the control of cisplatin-induced emesis. N Engl J Med 322 : 816–821
22. Milano S, Blower P, Romain D, Grelot L (1995) The piglet as a suitable animal model for studying the delayed phase of cisplatin-induced emesis. J Pharmcol Exp Ther 274 : 951–961
23. Moreno I, Rosell R, Abad A (1992) Comparison of three protracted antiemetic regimens for the control of delayed emesis in cisplatin -treated patients. Eur J Cancer [A] 28 : 1344–1347
24. Navari R, Madajewicz S, Anderson N, Tchekmedyian N, Whaley W, Garewal H, Beck T, Anderson E, Liddle R, Ossi M (1995) Oral ondansetron effectively controls cisplatin-induced delayed emesis. Proc Am Soc Clin Oncol 14 : 523
25. Passalacqua R, Cocconi G, Bella M, Monici L, Michiara M, Bandini N, Bacchi M (1992) Double-blind, randomized trial for the control of delayed emesis in patients receiving cisplatin: comparison of placebo vs. adrenocorticotropic hormone (ACTH). Ann Oncol 3 : 481–485
26. Pater JL, Lofters WS, Zrr B, Dempsey E, Walde D, Moquin J-P, Wilson K, Hoskins P, Guevin RM, Verma S, Navari R, Krook JE, Hainsworth J, Palmer M, Chin C (1997) The role of the $5HT_3$ antagonists ondansetron and dolasetron in the control of delayed onset nausea and vomiting in patients receiving moderately emetogenic chemotherapy. Ann Oncol 8 : 181–185
27. Research IGfA (1995) Ondansetron versus granisetron, both combined with dexamethasone, in the prevention of cisplatin-induced emesis. Ann Oncol 6 : 805–810
28. Research TIGfA (1997) Ondansetron versus metoclopramide, both combined with dexamethasone, in the prevention of cisplatin-induced delayed emesis. Clin Oncol 15 : 124–130
29. Rittenberg CN, Gralla RJ, Lettow LA, Cronin MD, Kardinal CG (1994) Combination antiemetic trials for delayed emesis (abstract). Proc Am Soc Clin Oncol 13 : 452
30. Roila F (1995) Dexamethasone, granisetron, or both for the prevention of nausea and vomiting during chemotherapy for cancer. N Engl J Med 332 : 1–5
31. Roila F, Bracarda S, Tonato M, Marangolo M, Bella M, Donati D, Cetto G, Del FA (1990) Ondansetron (GR38032) in the prophylaxis of acute and delayed cisplatin-induced emesis. Clin Oncol 2 : 268–272
32. Roila F, Boschetti E, Tonato M (1991) Predictive factors of delayed emesis in cisplatin treated patients and antiemetic activity and tolerability of metoclopramide or dexamethasone. A randomized single-blind study. Am J Clin Oncol 14 : 238–242
33. Rudd JA, Jordan CC, Naylor RJ (1996) The action of the tachykinin 1 receptor antagonist CP 99,994 to antagonise the acute and delayed emesis induced by cisplatin in the ferret. Br J Pharmacol
34. Rudd JA, Jordan CC, Naylor RJ (1994) Profiles of emetic action of cisplatin in the ferret: a potential model of acute and delayed emesis. Eur J Pharmacol 262 : R1–R2
35. Strum S, McDermed J, Abrahano-Umall R, Sanders P (1985) Management of cisplatin(DDP)-induced delayed-onset nausea (N) and vomiting (V): preliminary results with 2 drug regimens. Proc Am Soc Clin Oncol 4 : 263

Antiemetic Strategies for High-Dose Chemoradiotherapy-Induced Nausea and Vomiting

Thomas R. Spitzer, Steven M. Grunberg, Mario A. Dicato

ABSTRACT The treatment of nausea and vomiting in patients receiving high doses of irradiation and/or chemotherapeutic agents as preparation for hematopoietic stem cell transplantation is discussed.

Such patients have very high rates of both early and delayed emesis. Based on the available evidence, it is recommended that 5-HT_3 receptor antagonists be used to combat emesis in this setting. Continued research is also required to define the optimal antiemetic strategy for these patients.

Introduction

High-dose chemoradiotherapy as preparative therapy for hematopoietic stem cell transplantation provides a unique challenge in the prevention and management of emesis. Despite the widely held assumption that nausea and vomiting following high-dose chemoradiotherapy are more severe than with conventional-dose chemotherapy or radiotherapy, few published data exist to define the magnitude of this problem. Two analyses of emesis associated with fractionated (1320 cGy in 11 fractions) total-body irradiation (TBI) prior to high-dose chemotherapy have been performed [14, 15]. A total of 39 patients were analyzed, 29 of whom received combination non 5-HT_3 receptor antagonist antiemetic therapy, while the remaining ten were treated with placebo as part of a prospective double-blind randomized trial evaluating the efficacy of ondansetron in the prevention of TBI-induced emesis. Vomiting was universal among these 39 patients. In the 29 patients treated with combination antiemetic therapies, the peak number of emetic episodes occurred on the first day of treatment. Median number of emetic episodes over the 4-day treatment was five (range, one to 32). In nine of the ten placebo-treated patients, salvage antiemetic therapy was required on the first day of treatment. The natural history of emesis following high-dose chemotherapy is even less well established. A very high rate of early and delayed nausea and vomiting, however, has been documented in most published trials evaluating the toxicities of high-dose chemotherapy regimens for bone marrow transplantation.

Antiemetic Trials in Bone Marrow Transplantation

Total Body Irradiation

The recent availability of 5-HT$_3$ receptor antagonists and their demonstrated efficacy for prevention of chemotherapy- and radiation therapy-induced emesis have led to a series of clinical trials evaluating their role in the prevention of high-dose chemoradiotherapy-induced nausea and vomiting. Interpretation of the data from these studies has been hindered by several factors, however, including the retrospective nature of the majority of the studies, small patient numbers, variable antiemetic dosing regimens, and nonuniformity of the measurements of efficacy.

A series of retrospective analyses of the role of 5-HT$_3$ receptor antagonists for TBI-induced emesis have shown high (75–97%) complete or major responses to therapy [5, 7–9, 13]. In view of the historically high probability of nausea and vomiting after TBI, the results of these studies suggest that 5-HT$_3$ receptor antagonist were effective in the prevention of TBI-induced emesis.

Four prospective randomized trials have also evaluated the efficacy of 5-HT$_3$ receptor antagonists. The results of these trials are summarized in Table 1. Only one of the trials, however, involved high-dose chemotherapy given prior to TBI. In the study by Tiley et al., a prospective evaluation of a single 8-mg intravenous dose of ondansetron was evaluated in 20 patients receiving 110 mg/m^2 melphalan the day before single-dose TBI at 10.5 cGy [16]. All patients, however, also received phenobarbitone and corticosteroids for emetic control. Patients receiving ondansetron were found to have fewer emetic episodes than patients receiving placebo. Grant Prentice et al. evaluated the efficacy of granisetron against that of metoclopramide, dexamethasone, and lorazepam for the prevention of TBI-induced emesis [6]. All patients received chemotherapy including high-dose cyclophosphamide over 2 consecutive days. Chemotherapy was completed at least 66 h prior to TBI. Patients treated with granisetron had significantly improved control of vomiting and required less rescue therapy. In a prospective, randomized trial by Okamoto et al., comparing the antiemetic efficacy of granisetron and of ten different "standard" antiemetic regimens, 58 patients (43 of whom received TBI) undergoing conditioning for stem cell transplantation were evaluated [11]. Significantly fewer emetic episodes were observed in granisetron-treated patients.

We conducted a prospective, randomized, double-blind, placebo-controlled evaluation of ondansetron for the prevention of TBI-induced emesis [15]. Given our historical experience of universal vomiting with fractionated TBI (1320 cGy in 11 fractions over 4 days) despite combination antiemetic

Table 1 Prospective randomized trials of 5-HT$_3$ receptor antagonists in the prevention of TBI-induced emesis (*TBI* total-body irradiation, *sf* single fraction, *CY* cyclophosphamide, *OND* ondansetron, *GRA* granisetron, *MCP* metoclopramide, *DEX* dexamethasone, *LOR* lorazepam, *CR* complete response)

Center	Number of patients	Conditioning therapy	Drug/dose	Response/ outcome	Other	Reference
Royal Marsden London	20	MEL 110 mg/m2 → sf TBI 10.5 Gy	OND 8 mg i.v. before TBI vs placebo	↓ Emetic episodes (*p*=0.029) vs placebo		[16]
Georgetown, Washington, DC	20	TBI 13.2 Gy	OND 8 mg p.o. before each TBI dose vs placebo	↓ Emetic episodes (*p*=0.005), longer time to first emesis (*p*=0.003 vs placebo)	Rescue i.v. OND effective in 6/10 placebo-, 0/4 OND- treated patients	[15]
Royal Free Hospital, London	30	CY ± additional chemo → sf TBI 7.5 Gy	GRA 3 mg i.v. vs MCP 20 mg i.v. + DEX 6 mg/m^2 i.v. + LOR 2 mg. i.v.	↑ CR vs control, improved control of vomiting at 24 h, 7 days (*p*=0.001 and *p*=0.004)	Longer time to first emesis, ↓ requirement for rescue therapy vs control	[6]
Japan (multicenter)	43	Not specified	GRA 40 mcg/kg twice daily vs "standard" therapy	↓ Emetic episodes (*p*<0.001)		[10]

All patients also received phenobarbitone + corticosteroids

therapy, a placebo arm was included with rescue i.v. ondansetron administered in the event of emetic episodes comparable in number to our historical experience. The fractionated TBI regimen that we utilized, moreover, preceded high-dose chemotherapy, thus allowing for a more accurate assessment of the role of 5-HT$_3$ receptor antagonist therapy in prevention of TBI-induced emesis. Significantly fewer emetic episodes and a longer time-lapse to first emesis were observed in the ondansetron-treated group. The ten patients who received ondansetron included six who completed the entire 4-day study without the need for rescue antiemetic therapy. All ten placebo patients required rescue antiemetic therapy, nine of them on the first day of TBI. Rescue i.v. ondansetron therapy was found to be effective in control of

Table 2 Prospective randomized trials of 5-HT$_3$ receptor antagonists in the prevention of high-dose chemotherapy-induced emesis (*CY* cyclophosphamide, *BU* busulfan, *CI* continuous infusion, *MCP* metoclopramide, *DP* droperidol, *CP* chlorpromazine, *OND* ondansetron)

Center	Number of patients	Conditioning therapy	Drug/dose	Response outcome	Other	Reference
Seattle, Washington	30	CY	OND: low-vs high-dose[a] vs MCP/DP × 3 days	↓ Emetic episodes, ↓ nausea with OND; no advantage for high-dose OND	No correlation between OND levels and antiemetic efficacy	[1]
	30	BU/CY	OND: low-vs high-dose[a] vs MCP/DP × 7 days			
Florence, Italy	40	Multiple regimens	OND 8 mg i.v. followed by CI 1 mg/h vs CP 60 mg/m^2 per day by CI	No difference in antiemetic efficacy, control of nausea with OND	↓ Side effects (sedation, extra-pyramidal reactions)	[3]
Japan (multicenter)	15	Multiple regimens	GRA 40 mcg/kg twice daily vs "standard" therapy	Nonstatistically significant trend towards improved control of emesis		[11]

[a] Low dose: 0.1 mg/kg load, then 0.035 mg/kg per h by continuous infusion; high-dose: 0.2 mg/kg load, then 0.07 mg/kg per h by continuous infusion

emesis in six of the ten placebo-treated patients. None of the four patients who originally received oral ondansetron and subsequently required rescue therapy benefited from the rescue therapy. Ondansetron was well tolerated. No side effects were seen more frequently in the ondansetron-treated patients than in the placebo group.

High-Dose Chemotherapy

Limited data are also available to judge the efficacy of antiemetic strategies for the prevention of high-dose chemotherapy-induced nausea and vomiting. Several phase II trials have shown that 5-HT$_3$ receptor antagonists have significant activity in the control of early high-dose chemotherapy-induced emesis [2, 10, 12]. Two prospective, randomized trials evaluating the 5-HT$_3$

receptor antagonists are described in Table 2. Ondansetron was shown to be superior to metoclopramide and droperidol in a trial by Agura et al. at the Fred Hutchinson Cancer Research Center [1]. No improvement in emetic control was seen with "high"- versus "low"-dose ondansetron, and no correlation between ondansetron levels and antiemetic efficacy was observed. The designation of "high" versus "low" doses of ondansetron is, however, misleading. A 70-kg patient in the low-dose treatment group would have received approximately 63 mg of ondansetron in 24 h. In a study by Bosi et al., evaluating primarily high-dose chemotherapy-treated bone marrow transplant recipients, continuous infusional chlorpromazine was comparable to continuous infusional ondansetron in terms of antiemetic efficacy and control of nausea [3]. Side effects, particularly sedation and extrapyramidal reactions, however, were significantly less frequent in ondansetron-treated patients. In the trial by Okamoto et al., 15 patients received chemotherapy-only conditioning regimens [11]. No statistically significant difference in the control of emesis was observed between granisetron and standard antiemetic therapy.

Remaining Issues

While the efficacy of 5-HT$_3$ receptor antagonists in the prevention of acute nausea and vomiting after high-dose chemoradiotherapeutic preparative regimens for bone marrow transplantation has been established, there is considerably less published experience, both from the standpoint of description of the natural history and from that of the impact of therapeutic maneuvers on its incidence, or the severity of delayed nausea and vomiting. In our experience, however, delayed nausea and vomiting are nearly universal following bone marrow transplantation and appear to be independent of the antiemetic regimen used during the transplant preparative regimen. Delayed emesis, moreover, is influenced by multiple confounding variables, including infusion of cryopreserved stem cells, and concomitant medications (antibiotics, cyclosporine, opiates, etc).

While 5-HT$_3$ receptor antagonists are effective in the prevention of early chemoradiotherapy-induced nausea and vomiting, antiemetic protection is incomplete. Thus combination antiemetic drug strategies are often employed. There are presently insufficient data to support the use of any one combination regimen rather than another.

The choice of regimen, moreover, is influenced by several factors, including concomitant chemoradiotherapy-induced toxicities (e.g., diarrhea limiting the use of metoclopramide) and concerns about pharmacokinetic interactions that might alter chemotherapy metabolism and efficacy (e.g., possible interference with cyclophosphamide metabolism by dexamethasone).

Anecdotal evidence suggests the possibility of a dose-response relationship for the 5-HT$_3$ receptor antagonists in the prevention of TBI-induced emesis. The study by Agura et al. showed that relatively high doses of ondansetron were effective in the prevention of high-dose chemotherapy-induced emesis. The success of 5-HT$_3$ receptor antagonist antiemetic regimens in preventing acute emesis associated with transplant conditioning regimens thus validates our ability to stay on the plateau portion of the dose-response curve with appropriate dosing. However, this success should also serve as a warning that dose deescalation of antiemetics, which has been used successfully with standard chemotherapeutic regimens [4], should be approached with caution in a setting where the dose-response curve may be shifted to the right and de-escalation to a point below the threshold value could more easily occur.

Recommendations

1. Based on several randomized studies, we recommend the use of 5-HT$_3$ receptor antagonists for the prevention of TBI-induced emesis. Available evidence suggests that high-dose 5-HT$_3$ receptor antagonists also have efficacy for the prevention of acute emesis induced by high-dose chemotherapeutic conditioning regimens.

2. Further studies are necessary to determine the optimal dosage and timing of 5-HT$_3$ receptor antagonists to establish whether combination antiemetic treatment is more effective than 5-HT$_3$ receptor antagonists alone.

3. No therapy has been definitely known to alter the incidence or severity of delayed high-dose chemoradiotherapy-induced nausea and vomiting. Clinical trials evaluating new antiemetic therapies will be necessary.

References

1. Agura ED, Cleveland Brown M, Schaffer R, Donaldson G, Shen DD (1995) Anti-emetic efficacy and pharmacokinetics of intravenous ondansetron infusion during chemotherapy conditioning for bone marrow transplant. Bone Marrow Transplant 16 : 213–222
2. Barbounis V, Koumakis G, Vassilomanolakis M, Hatzichristou H, Tsousis S, Efremidis AP (1995) A phase II study of ondansetron as antiemetic prophylaxis in patients receiving high-dose polychemotherapy and stem cell transplantation 3 : 301–306
3. Bosi A, Guidi S, Messori A et al (1993) Ondansetron versus chlorpromazine for preventing emesis in born marrow transplant recipients: a double-blind randomized study. J Chemother 5 : 191–196

4. Di Piro CV, Sanal SM, Harkness KT et al (1996) The anti-emetic efficacy of intravenous ondansetron at conventional versus low dose in women with early stage breast cancer. Proc Am Soc Clin Oncol 15 : 540
5. Feuvret L, Jammet P, Campana F, Cosset JM, Fourquet A (1994) Interet du granisetron dans la prevention des troubles digestifs lors des irradiations corporelles totales. Bull Cancer/Radiother 81 : 41–44
6. Grant Prentice H, Cunningham S, Gandhi L, Cunningham J, Collis C, Harmon MD (1995) Granisetron in the prevention of irradiation-induced emesis. Bone Marrow Transplant 15 : 445–448
7. Hewitt M, Cornish J, Pamphilon D, Oakhill A (1991) Effective emetic control during conditioning of children for bone marrow transplantation using ondansetron, a 5-HT$_3$ receptor antagonist. Bone Marrow Transplant 7 : 431–433
8. Hunter AE, Prentice HG, Pothecary K et al (1991) Granisetron, a selective 5-HT$_3$ receptor antagonist, for the prevention of radiation induced emesis during total body irradiation. Bone Marrow Transplant 7 : 439–441
9. Jurgens H, McQuade B (1992) Ondansetron as prophylaxis for chemotherapy and radiotherapy induced emesis in children. Oncology 49 : 279–285
10. Koleck P, Wachowiak J, Beshari SE (1993) Ondansetron as an effective drug in prophylaxis of chemotherapy-induced emesis in children. Acta Haematol Pol 24 : 115–122
11. Okamoto S, Takahashi S, Tanosaki R et al (1996) Granisetran in the prevention of vomiting induced by conditioning for stem cell transplantation: a prospective randomized study. Bone Marrow Transplant 17 : 679–683
12. Or R, Drakos P, Nagler A, Naparstek E, Kapelushnik J, Cass Y (1994) The anti-emetic efficacy and tolerability of tropisetron in patients with high-dose chemotherapy (with and without total body irradiation) prior to bone marrow transplantation. Support Care Cancer 2 : 245–248
13. Schwella N, Konig V, Schwerdtfeger R et al (1994) Ondansetron for efficient emesis control during total body irradiation. Bone Marrow Transplant 13 : 169–171
14. Spitzer TR, Deeg HJ, Torrisi J et al (1990) Total body irradiation induced emesis is universal after small dose fractions (120 cGy) and is not cumulative dose related. Proc ASCO 9 : 14
15. Spitzer TR, Bryson JC, Cirenza E et al (1994) Randomized double-blind, placebo-controlled evaluation of oral ondansetron in the prevention of nausea and vomiting associated with fractionated total-body irradiation. J Clin Oncol 12 : 2432–2435
16. Tiley C, Powles R, Catalano J et al (1992) Results of a double blind placebo controlled study of ondansetron as an antiemetic during total body irradiation in patients undergoing bone marrow transplantation. Leuk Lymph 7 : 317–321

Consensus Proposal for 5-HT$_3$ Antagonists in the Prevention of Acute Emesis Related to Highly Emetogenic Chemotherapy

Dose, Schedule, and Route of Administration

David R. Gandara, Fausto Roila, David Warr, Martin J. Edelman, Edith A. Perez, Richard J. Gralla

ABSTRACT Selective antagonists to the type 3 serotonin receptor (5-HT$_3$) in combination with corticosteroids are now considered the standard of care for the prevention of emesis from moderately to highly emetogenic chemotherapy. Here we address issues of optimal dose, schedule, and route of administration of four currently available selectable 5-HT$_3$ antagonists. This paper utilizes an evidence-based medicine approach to the literature regarding this class of drugs, emphasizing the results of large, randomized, controlled trials to make formal recommendations concerning optimal use of this important new class of antiemetic agents. We conclude that for each drug there is a plateau in therapeutic efficacy at a definable dose level above which further dose escalation does not improve outcome. Furthermore, a single dose is as effective as multiple doses or continuous infusion, and finally, emerging data demonstrate that the oral route is equally efficacious as the intravenous route of administration, even with highly emetogenic chemotherapy.

Introduction

The development of selective antagonists to the 5-hydroxytryptamine (5-HT$_3$) receptor has revolutionized the therapeutic approach to chemotherapy-induced emesis (CIE) [21, 28, 49]. These agents, in combination with corticosteroids, have become a new standard of care for moderately to highly emetogenic chemotherapy. The four selective 5-HT$_3$ antagonists that have completed clinical testing (ondansetron, granisetron, tropisetron, and dolasetron) differ considerably in biological properties such as receptor specificity, potency, and plasma half-life [2, 50]. Nevertheless, each has demonstrated relatively equivalent efficacy in the prevention of CIE in a wide variety of clinical settings. As a class, these agents are characterized by an excellent side effect profile and a broad therapeutic index. Despite these advantages and widespread clinical use, a number of controversies and uncertainties regarding the optimal use of these agents in day-to-day clinical practice persist.

This discussion will address issues of dose, schedule, and route of administration of the four selective 5-HT$_3$ antagonists in the prevention of acute emesis induction by moderately to highly emetogenic chemotherapy, based on an assessment of the best available literature. Rigorously designed double-blind randomized trials (phase III) of sufficient sample size were considered to offer the most valid evidence, whereas uncontrolled clinical trials, observation, and retrospective analysis each provided weaker evidence in support of a proposed recommendation. This approach is consistent with recent recommendations regarding evidence-based medicine [17]. Selected studies forming the basis for recommendations for each agent are summarized in selected references. The "no emesis" rate during the initial 24-h observation period (acute emesis) was selected as an appropriate therapeutic end point universally reported in the trials under consideration.

In this presentation, we have formulated a hypothesis regarding each of the three issues to be addressed (dose, schedule, and route), summarized data in support of and contradictory to the stated hypothesis, reached conclusions based on the balance of evidence, and made recommendations for use of these agents in clinical practice.

Dose

Hypothesis

Despite preclinical differences, the 5-HT$_3$ antagonists are characterized clinically by: (1) a threshold effect for response, (2) a modest dose-response curve, and (3) a plateau in therapeutic efficacy extending over a severalfold range in dose.

If valid, the therapeutic implications are considerable; they can be summarized as follows: (1) more is not necessarily better, and (2) breakthrough emesis may be due to other mediators and/or receptors and not due to inadequate 5-HT$_3$ receptor blockade [27, 61].

If this hypothesis regarding dose is valid, how then do we justify the existing uncertainties regarding optimal dose of the available 5-HT$_3$ antagonists? For two agents in particular (ondansetron and granisetron), there is wide variability in the "approved" single dose level for prevention of acute emesis from highly emetogenic chemotherapy. If approved single dose levels are contrasted between the United States and Europe, there is an apparent paradox: in the United States the approved dose of ondansetron (32 mg or approximately 0.45 mg/kg) is fourfold that in Europe (8 mg), while for granisetron, exactly the opposite is true (10 mcg/kg vs 3 mg or 40 mcg/kg). Is it possible that the lower dose level for each agent is already on the therapeutic plateau, or do these lower doses fall somewhere along the dose-response curve?

In view of the above considerations, analysis of best available literature regarding dose was performed for each of the four 5-HT$_3$ antagonists which have completed clinical testing. Both dose-response studies of individual agents and comparative trials between agents were considered. Study designs incorporating overlapping issues of schedule are addressed in the next section on this topic.

Highly Emetogenic Chemotherapy

Cisplatin-based chemotherapy at doses over 50 mg/m^2 serves as a model for highly emetogenic chemotherapy. Randomized studies have generally demonstrated superiority of 5-HT$_3$ antagonists over high-dose intravenous metoclopramide, the previous standard, for prevention of acute CIE from cisplatin [10, 13, 25, 43, 59]. Furthermore, the addition of dexamethasone has consistently improved efficacy compared to a 5-HT$_3$ antagonist alone, establishing this combination as a standard for patients receiving cisplatin-based therapy [29, 53]. Dose-ranging studies of these agents generally demonstrate evidence of a dose-response curve consistent with the hypothesis stated above [22, 23, 37, 39, 45, 53, 60, 62, 63]. There are conflicting data regarding the optimal single dose of ondansetron for prevention of acute CIE from cisplatin. While a study published by Beck et al. led to the conclusion that a 32-mg dose was superior to 8 mg, particularly in patients receiving high-dose cisplatin (>100 mg/m^2), a similarly designed study by Seynaeve showed that the 8-mg dose was equally effective [3, 57]. In both studies, single-dose administration was equivalent to other approved dose schedules (see below). Further evidence in support of a single 8-mg ondansetron dose comes from the studies of the Italian Group for Antiemetic Research (IGAR) and from Ruff, an 8-mg dose showing equal efficacy to either a 32-mg dose level or 3 mg of granisetron, respectively [32, 56].

For granisetron, the balance of evidence from both dose-response studies of this agent and comparative trials against ondansetron supports a recommended dosing level of 10 mcg/kg [45, 46, 53, 59]. The dose-ranging studies of Navari and Riviere suggest that dose levels of 2 or 5 mcg/kg are suboptimal, while there is a relative plateau above 10 mcg/kg, with slightly higher, but probably clinically insignificant, "no emesis" rates at 40 mcg/kg [45, 53]. The comparative trial by Navari adds further support in favor of the 10-mcg/kg dose, with identical "no emesis" rates for 10 vs 40 mcg/kg in comparison to an approved and effective multiple dose schedule of ondansetron (0.15 mg/kg × 3) [46].

The dose-ranging study of Van Belle and the comparative trial by Marty both support a 5-mg single-dose administration of tropisetron as effective in highly emetogenic cisplatin-based chemotherapy, with the study of Van Belle suggesting no further improvement in efficacy at dose levels up to 40 mg [44, 63].

Initial dose-ranging studies of dolasetron did not clearly define the lowest effective dose, while the subsequent comparative trial of Hesketh supports a dose level of 1.8 mg/kg as effective, with no evidence of clinically significant improvement in efficacy at 2.4 mg/kg [31, 39, 62].

Since the emetogenic potential of cisplatin is dose related, the emesis from regimens in which cisplatin is given at low daily doses differs in severity and pattern from that induced by high-dose cisplatin. Several comparative studies have evaluated the antiemetic efficacy of the 5-HT$_3$ receptor antagonists in this setting and have demonstrated equal or superior activity to high-dose metoclopramide or alizapride [7, 20, 58]. These trials have also shown that antiemetic efficacy of 5-HT$_3$ antagonists is improved by the addition of a corticosteroid, similar to results with high-dose cisplatin [18, 47, 52].

Moderately Emetogenic Chemotherapy

Intravenous cyclophosphamide, doxorubicin, epirubicin, and carboplatin, alone or in combination, have been used as the emetogenic challenge in studies evaluating the efficacy of 5-HT$_3$ antagonists in moderately emetogenic chemotherapy. Corticosteroids, with or without other agents, have been the principal antiemetics used in patients receiving this type of therapy. Comparative studies of 5-HT$_3$ receptor antagonists have shown them to be superior in antiemetic activity to metoclopramide [1, 6, 9, 35, 41, 60], alizapride [11, 14], and phenothiazines [42, 48, 64]. When compared with dexamethasone alone, the 5-HT$_3$ receptor antagonists show equivalent, but not superior, antiemetic efficacy [33, 34]. Furthermore, a trial by the IGAR demonstrated that the combination of granisetron plus dexamethasone was superior to dexamethasone alone or granisetron alone (complete protection from acute vomiting in 93%, 71%, and 72%, respectively) [33]. Thus the combination of a corticosteroid and a 5-HT$_3$ antagonist appears to provide optimal antiemetic therapy in patients receiving this type of chemotherapy. Oral 5-HT$_3$ antagonists are appropriate in this setting, and there is a large body of literature to support this route of administration, as discussed later.

Appropriate dose selection of oral 5-HT$_3$ antagonists for moderately emetogenic chemotherapy has been problematic, in part due to interactive issues of schedule. Early trials of oral ondansetron utilized a multiple-dose schedule, and these regimens have since become standard practice. Informative trials regarding oral ondansetron dosing in this clinical setting include those of Beck and Cubbedu, demonstrating a plateau in efficacy at a total daily dose of 12 mg (4 mg TID), and a large trial by Dicato et al., in which 8 mg ondansetron twice daily was equivalent to 8 mg three times daily [4, 12, 15].

Table 1 Recommendations: 5-HT$_3$ antagonists in cisplatin chemotherapy-induced emesis

Agent	Daily dose	Schedule	Route	Consensus	Confidence
Ondansetron	8 mg	Single dose	i.v.	High	High
Granisetron	10 mcg/kg	Single dose	i.v.	High	High
	2 mg	Single dose	p.o.	High	Moderate
Tropisetron	5 mg	Single dose	i.v.	High	Moderate
Dolasetron	1.8 mg/kg	Single dose	i.v.	High	High

Table 2 Recommendations: oral 5-HT$_3$ antagonists in moderately emetogenic chemotherapy

Agent	Daily dose	Schedule	Consensus	Confidence
Ondansetron	12–16 mg	t.i.d. or b.i.d.	High	High
Granisetron	2 mg	Each day (or b.i.d.)	High	High
Tropisetron	_a	_a	_a	_a
Dolasetron	100–200 mg	Each day	High	Moderate

a Insufficient data available

Thus a daily dose of 12–16 mg represents a fully effective dose level of oral ondansetron in moderately emetogenic chemotherapy.

An oral dose-ranging trial of granisetron reported by Bleiberg et al. [5] compared 0.25 mg b.i.d., 0.5 mg b.i.d., 1.0 mg b.i.d., and 2 mg b.i.d.. All dose levels were superior to 0.25 mg, and there was no increase in efficacy above the 1.0 mg b.i.d. level. Similar results for 7-day efficacy were obtained by Hacking et al. [24]. As discussed below in the section on Schedule, a subsequent trial demonstrated equivalence of 1.0 mg b.i.d. and 2.0 mg as a single dose. Therefore, the most appropriate total daily oral dose of granisetron appears to be 2 mg. Studies by Rubenstein and Fauser have defined effective oral dose levels of dolasetron as 100–200 mg administered as a single dose [55]. There is insufficient information at present to allow us to make recommendations on the oral dosing of tropisetron.

In general, these dosing recommendations for oral administration of 5-HT$_3$ antagonists result in dosing ratios of 1.5–2:1 relative to the recommended single dose levels when they are given i.v. (Tables 1, 2). These dosing recommendations appear reasonable in view of the reported oral bioavailability of approximately 60% for 5-HT$_3$ antagonists as a drug class [21, 49].

Conclusions

Effective dose levels have been established for each of the four 5-HT$_3$ antagonists in both moderately and highly emetogenic chemotherapy. The lowest fully effective dose of each agent should be used in clinical practice.

Schedule

Hypothesis

If given at an effective dose level, a single dose provides adequate 5-HT$_3$ blockade for prevention of acute emesis. If valid, the implications regarding schedule of administration (for acute CIE) are as follows: (1) administration of multiple doses is unnecessary, and (2) breakthrough emesis during the acute phase may be related to other mediators/receptors. If a model for schedule is developed based on this hypothesis, then multiple doses will only provide a better therapeutic outcome if the initial dose were suboptimal, or if optimal therapeutic efficacy were dependent on the either plasma half-life or duration of receptor blockade during the acute phase.

Highly Emetogenic Chemotherapy

As discussed below, there is substantial evidence in support of the proposed hypothesis regarding schedule. Schedule effects are best assessed in studies of ondansetron, the first 5-HT$_3$ antagonist developed. Early clinical trials of i.v. ondansetron in cisplatin chemotherapy explored a variety of schedule-related issues, including variable dosing intervals, number of doses, and schedules incorporating continuous infusion [29, 38]. In general, these studies demonstrated that shortening the dosing interval or increasing the number of doses did not improve efficacy. A continuous infusion schedule following an 8 mg i.v. bolus was also found to be effective [43]. However, as demonstrated in the subsequent studies of Beck and Seynaeve, multiple-dose administration or continuous infusion schedules of ondansetron proved no more effective than single-dose administration [3, 57]. Based on these observations, development of the three other 5-HT$_3$ antagonists quickly evolved into determining optimal levels for i.v. single-dose administration.

Moderately Emetogenic Chemotherapy

Oral administration of 5-HT$_3$ antagonists by multiple-dose schedules has been extensively studied and is highly effective in the prevention of acute emesis from moderately emetogenic chemotherapy regimens. However, it remains unclear whether multiple doses are superior to a fully effective single dose, since few studies have addressed this issue in moderately emetogenic chemotherapy. In a randomized double-blind trial, however, oral granisetron at a single dose of 2 mg was equally effective as a standard divided-dose schedule (1 mg twice daily), with "no emesis" rates of 82% and 77%, respectively [16]. In a similar fashion, a trial by Kaizer et al. showed no difference in efficacy of 16 mg ondansetron i.v. as a single dose versus 8 mg i.v. plus 8 mg p.o. 12 h later [36]. These findings are compatible with the hypothesis that a fully effective dose of a 5-HT$_3$ antagonist need be administered only once in the prevention of acute CIE, regardless of the emetogenic challenge.

Conclusions

Single-dose intravenous administration is equally efficacious to multiple-dose or continuous infusion schedules and is the preferred schedule of administration for prevention of acute emesis from highly emetogenic chemotherapy. For moderately emetogenic chemotherapy, few studies have compared single versus multiple oral doses. However, when direct comparisons have been performed, oral single-dose administration at the appropriate dose level has been equivalent to multiple doses and is an acceptable alternative.

Route

Hypothesis

Oral administration of the 5-HT$_3$ antagonists is equally efficacious as intravenous (i.v.) administration.

Obviously, the most important implication of this hypothesis, if valid, is that since oral administration is generally less expensive and less resource intensive, this route may be preferable. There are three qualifiers to be considered in regard to this hypothesis: (1) there should be good oral drug bioavailability, (2) there must be an intact gastrointestinal tract to ensure absorption, and (3) compliance must be assured.

Moderately to Highly Emetogenic Chemotherapy

As a class, 5-HT$_3$ antagonists exhibit good drug bioavailability when administered by the oral route. While oral use is of proven efficacy for moderately emetogenic chemotherapy, to date there has been very little information regarding oral dosing for CIE from cisplatin. However, there is now emerging support for the administration of selective 5-HT$_3$ antagonists by the oral route even in the prevention of cisplatin-induced emesis. In a study by Heron [26], a standard combination of high-dose i.v. metoclopramide plus dexamethasone was compared with 1 mg oral granisetron alone (b.i.d.) or oral granisetron plus dexamethasone in cisplatin-treated patients. The "no emesis" rates were: oral granisetron (56%), metoclopramide/dexamethasone (52%), and granisetron/dexamethasone (66%). In a recently completed phase III trial, oral granisetron (2 mg) was compared with i.v. ondansetron (32 mg) in patients receiving cisplatin-based (>60 mg/m^2) chemotherapy [20]. Concomitant dexamethasone (10–20 mg) was administered in 80% of patients. Rates of total control (no nausea, no emesis, and no rescue) were similar in the two treatment arms, 55% with oral granisetron and 58% with i.v. ondansetron, while the "no emesis" rate was marginally higher with ondansetron (67%) than with granisetron (61%). Although a single study, this was a large ($n = 1054$) and well-designed trial (double-blind, stratified by gender), and the results support the use of oral 5-HT$_3$ antagonists, even in cisplatin-treated patients. Adding further support is a similarly designed comparative trial by Perez et al. of oral granisetron versus i.v. ondansetron with moderately emetogenic chemotherapy, which also demonstrated equal efficacy for these two routes of administration [51].

Conclusions

Assuming an intact gastrointestinal tract to ensure absorption, and good compliance, the oral route is an acceptable alternative to intravenous administration. For moderately emetogenic chemotherapy, oral administration of 5-HT$_3$ antagonists is well established, usually in combination with a corticosteroid. In cisplatin-induced CIE, preliminary support exists for granisetron at a 2-mg oral dose in combination with dexamethasone.

Overall Summary and Recommendations

Based on analysis of best available literature regarding dose, schedule, and route of 5-HT$_3$ antagonists for prevention of acute emesis from moderately to highly emetogenic chemotherapy, summary conclusions are as follows:
1. Dose: It is recommended that a fully effective dose level of each agent be administered. Cost-effectiveness dictates that this be the minimum fully effective dose. However, underdosing these agents which are characterized by an excellent side effect profile and high therapeutic index, should be avoided.

       Level of consensus: High
       Level of confidence: High

2. Schedule: If given at an effective dose level, it is unnecessary to administer multiple intravenous doses or deliver these agents as a continuous infusion.

>   Level of consensus: High
>   Level of confidence: High

3. Route: Administration of 5-HT$_3$ antagonists by the oral route is well established for moderately emetogenic chemotherapy. Preliminary data suggest that the oral route is also equivalent to intravenous administration, even in patients receiving high-dose cisplatin.

>   Level of consensus: High
>   Level of confidence: High

4. Overall: The combination of a 5HT$_3$ antagonist plus a corticosteroid represents the standard of care for patients receiving moderate to highly emetogenic chemotherapy.

>   Level of consensus: High
>   Level of confidence: High

Consensus recommendations for each specific agent in the prevention of acute emesis from highly and moderately emetogenic chemotherapy are presented in Tables 1 and 2, respectively. These recommendations represent an analysis of best available literature, using an evidence-based medicine approach, as well as reflecting the input of discussants and participants during this consensus conference.

In conclusion, the 5-HT$_3$ antagonists have substantially improved the management of CIE, and these agents in combination with corticosteroids can be considered the standard of care in patients receiving moderately to highly emetogenic chemotherapy. Nevertheless, many patients continue to experience CIE, often related to late breakthrough or delayed emesis. It is likely that the majority of these episodes are mediated through non-5-HT$_3$-induced mechanisms. Further improvements in therapy await better definition of the underlying pathophysiology of these events and development of selective antagonists to the involved receptors.

References

1. Anderson H, Thatcher N, Howell A et al (1994) Tropisetron compared with a metoclopramide-based regimen in the prevention of chemotherapy induced nausea and vomiting. Eur J Cancer 30 : 610–615
2. Andrews PLR, Davis CJ (1993) The mechanism of emesis induced by anti-cancer therapies. In: Andrews PLR, Sanger GJ (eds) Emesis in anticancer therapy, mechanisms and treatment. Chapman & Hall, London, pp 14–17

3. Beck TM, Hesketh PJ, Madajewicz S, Navari RM, Pendergrass K, Lester KP, Kish JA, Murphy WK, Hainsworth JD, Gandara DR, Bricker LJ, Keller AM, Mortimer J, Galvin DV, House KW, Bryson JC (1992) Stratified, randomized, double-blind comparison of intravenous ondansetron administered as a multiple-dose regimen versus two single-dose regimens in the prevention of cisplatin-induced nausea and vomiting. J Clin Oncol 10 : (12); 1969–1975

4. Beck TM, Ciociola AA, Jones SE, Harvey WH, Tchekmedyian NS, Chiang A, Galvin D, Hart NE (1993) Efficacy of oral ondansetron in the prevention of emesis in outpatients receiving cyclophosphamide-based chemotherapy. Ann Intern Med 118 : 407–413

5. Bleiberg HH, Spielmann M, Falkson G et al (1995) Antiemetic treatment with oral granisetron in patients receiving moderately emetogenic chemotherapy: dose ranging study. Clin Therapeutics 17 : 38–51

6. Bonneterre J, Chevalier B, Metz R et al (1990) A randomized double-blind comparison of ondansetron and metoclopramide in the prophylaxis of emesis induced by cyclophosphamide, fluorouracil and doxorubicin or epirubicin chemotherapy. J Clin Oncol 8 : 1063–1069

7. Bremer K, on behalf of the Granisetron Study Group (1992) A single-blind study of the efficacy and safety of intravenous granisetron compared with alizapride plus dexamethasone in the prophylaxis and control of emesis in patients receiving 5-day cytostatic therapy. Eur J Cancer [A] 28 : 1018–1022

8. Buser KS, Joss RA, Piquet D et al (1993) Oral ondansetron in the prophylaxis of nausea and vomiting induced by cyclophosphamide, methotrexate and 5-fluorouracil (CMF) in women with breast cancer. Results of a prospective, randomized, double-blind, placebo controlled study. Ann Oncol 4 : 475–479

9. Campora E, Giudici S, Merlini L et al (1994) Ondansetron and dexamethasone versus standard combination antiemetic therapy. Am J Clin Oncol (CCT) 17 : 522–526

10. Chevalier B (1990) Efficacy and safety of granisetron compared with high-dose metoclopramide plus dexamethasone in patients receiving high-dose cisplatin in a single-blind study. Eur J Cancer 26 [Suppl 1] : 33–36

11. Clavel M, Bonneterre J, d'Allens H, French Ondansetron Study Group (1995) Oral ondansetron in the prevention of chemotherapy-induced emesis in breast cancer patients. Eur J Cancer [A] 31 : 15–19

12. Cubeddu LX, Pendergrass K, Ryan T, York M, Burton G, Meshad M, Galvin D, Ciociola AA (1994) Efficacy of oral ondansetron, a selective antagonist of $5HT_3$ receptors, in the treatment of nausea and vomiting associated with cyclophosphamide-based chemotherapies. Ondansetron Study Group. Am J Clin Oncol 17 : 137–146

13. De Mulder PHM, Seynaeve C, Vermorken JB et al (1990) Ondansetron (GR38032F) versus high dose metoclopramide in the prophylaxis of acute and delayed cisplatin-induced nausea and vomiting. Ann Intern Med 113 : 834–840

14. De Nigris A, Paladini G, Giosa F et al (1994) Tropisetron (Navoban) compared with alizapride in the control of emesis induced by cyclophosphamide-containing regimens. Eur J Cancer [A] 30 : 1902–1903

15. Dicato MA (1991) Oral treatment with ondansetron in the outpatient setting. Eur J Cancer 27 [Suppl 1] : 518–519

16. Ettinger DS, Eisenberg PD, Fitts D, Friedman C, Wilson-Lynch K, Yocom K (1996) A double-blind comparison of the efficacy of two dose regimens of oral granisetron in preventing acute emesis in patient receiving moderately emetogenic chemotherapy. Cancer 78 : 144–151

17. Evidence-Based Medicine Working Group (1992) Evidence-based medicine: a new approach to teaching the practice of medicine. JAMA 268 : 420–425

18. Fox SM, Einhorn LH, Cox E, et al (1993) Ondansetron vs ondansetron, dexamethasone, and chlorpromazine in the prevention of nausea and vomiting associated with multiple-day cisplatin chemotherapy. J Clin Oncol 11 : 2391–2395

19. Gralla RJ, Popovic W, Strupp J, Culleton V, Preston A, Friedman C (1997) Can an oral antiemetic regimen be as effective as intravenous treatment against cisplatin: results of a 1054 patient randomized study of oral granisetron versus IV ondansetron. Proc Am Soc Clin Oncol 16 : 52a (#178)

20. Granisetron Study Group (1993) The antiemetic efficacy and safety of granisetron compared with metoclopramide plus dexamethasone in patients receiving fractionated chemotherapy over 5 days. J Cancer Res Clin Oncol 199 : 555–559

21. Grunberg SM, Hesketh PJ (1993) Control of chemotherapy-induced emesis. N Engl J Med 329 : 1790–1796

22. Grunberg SM, Stevenson LL, Russell CA et al (1989) Dose ranging phase I study of the serotonin antagonist GR38032F for prevention of cisplatin-induced nausea and vomiting. J Clin Oncol 7 : 1137–1141

23. Grunberg SM, Lane M, Lester EP, Sridhar KS, Monimer J, Murphy W, Sanderson PE (1993) Randomized double blind comparison of three dose levels of intravenous ondansetron in the prevention of cisplatin-induced emesis. Cancer Chemother Pharmacol 32 : 268–272

24. Hacking A (1992) Oral granisetron – simple and effective. A preliminary report. Granisetron Study Group. Eur J Cancer [Suppl 1] : 28–32

25. Hainsworth J, Harvey W, Pendergrass K et al (1991) A single-blind comparison of intravenous ondansetron, a selective antagonist, with intravenous metoclopramide in the prevention of nausea and vomiting associated with high-dose cisplatin chemotherapy. J Clin Oncol 9 : 721–728

26. Heron JF (1995) Single-agent oral granisetron for the prevention of acute cisplatin-induced emesis: a double-blind, randomized comparison with granisetron plus dexamethasone and high-dose metoclopramide plus dexamethasone. Semin Oncol 22 [Suppl 10] : 24–30

27. Herrstedt J (1996) New perspectives in antiemetic treatment. Support Care Cancer 4 : 416–419

28. Hesketh PJ, Gandara DR (1991) Serotonin antagonists: a new class of antiemetic agents. J Natl Cancer Inst 83 : 613–620

29. Hesketh PJ, Murphy WK, Lester EP, Gandara DR, Khojasteh A, Tapazoglou E, Sartiano GP, White DR, Werner K, Chubb JM (1989) GR 38032F (GR-C507/75): a novel compound effective in the prevention of acute cisplatin-induced emesis. J Clin Oncol 7 : 700–705

30. Hesketh PJ, Harvey WH, Harker WG et al (1994) A randomized, double-blind comparison of intravenous ondansetron alone and in combination with intravenous dexamethasone in the prevention of high-dose cisplatin-induced emesis. J Clin Oncol 12 : 596–600

31. Hesketh P, Navari R, Grote T, Gralla R, Hainsworth J, Kris M, Anthony L, Khojasteh A, Tapazoglou E, Benedict C, Hahne W, for the Dolasetron Comparative Chemotherapy-induced Emesis Prevention Group (1996) Double-blind, randomized comparison of the antiemetic efficacy of intravenous dolasetron mesylate and intravenous ondansetron in the prevention of acute cisplatin-induced emesis in patients with cancer. J Clin Oncol 14 : 2242–2249

32. Italian Group for Antiemetic Research (1995) Ondansetron versus granisetron, both combined with dexamethasone, in the prevention of cisplatin-induced emesis. Ann Oncol 6 : 805–810

33. Italian Group for Antiemetic Research (1995) Dexamethasone, granisetron, or both for the prevention of nausea and vomiting during chemotherapy for cancer. N Engl J Med 332 : 1–5

34. Jones AL, Hill AS, Soukop M et al (1991) Comparison of ondansetron and dexamethasone in the prophylaxis of emesis induced by moderately emetogenic chemotherapy. Lancet 338 : 483–487

35. Kaasa S, Kvaloy S, Dicato MA et al (1990) A comparison of ondansetron with metoclopramide in the prophylaxis of chemotherapy-induced nausea and vomiting: a randomized, double-blind study. Eur J Cancer 26 : 311–314

36. Kaizer L, Warr D, Hoskins P, Latreille J, Lofters W, Yau J, Palmer M, Zee B, Levy M, Pater J (1994) Effect of schedule and maintenance on the antiemetic efficacy of ondansetron combined with dexamethasone in acute and delayed nausea and emesis in patients receiving moderately emetogenic chemotherapy: a phase III trial by the National Cancer Institute of Canada Clinical Trials Group. J Clin Oncol 12 : 1050–1057

37. Kris MG, Gralla RJ, Clark RA et al (1988) Dose-ranging evaluation of the serotonin antagonist GRC507/75 (GR38032F) when used as an antiemetic in patients receiving anticancer chemotherapy. J Clin Oncol 6 : 659–662

38. Kris MG, Gralla RJ, Clark RA, Tyson LB (1989) Phase II trials of the serotonin antagonist GR38032F for the control of vomiting caused by cisplatin. J Natl Cancer Institute 81 : 42–46

39. Kris MG, Grunberg SM, Gralla RJ, Baltzer L, Zarentsky SA, Litsey D, Tyson LB, Schmidt L, Hahne WF (1994) Dose-ranging evaluation of the serotonin antagonist dolasetron mesylate in patients receiving high-dose cisplatin. J Clin Oncol 12 : 1045–1049

40. Levitt M, Warr D, Yell L et al 1993) Ondansetron compared with dexamethasone and metoclopramide as antiemetics in the chemotherapy of breast cancer with cyclophosphamide, methotrexate and fluorouracil. N Engl J Med 328 : 1081–1084

41. Marschner NW, Adler M, Nagel GA et al (1991) Double-blind randomized trial of the antiemetic efficacy and safety of ondansetron and metoclopramide in advanced breast cancer patients treated with epirubicin and cyclophosphamide. Eur J Cancer 27 : 1137–1140

42. Marty M, on behalf of the Granisetron Study Group (1990) A comparative study of the use of granisetron, a selective 5HT3 antagonist, versus a standard antiemetic regimen of chlorpromazine plus dexamethasone in the treatment of cytostatic-induced emesis. Eur J Cancer 26 [Suppl 1] : 28–32

43. Marty M, Pouillart P, Scholl S (1990) Comparison of the 5-hydroxytryptamine (serotonin) antagonist ondansetron (GR 38032F) with high-dose metaclopromide in the control of cisplatin-induced emesis. N Engl J Med 322 : 816–821

44. Marty M, Kleisbauer J-P, Fournet P, Vergnenegro A, Caries P, Loria-Kanza Y, Simonetta C, Bruijn KM de, the French Navoban Study Group (1995) Is Navoban (tropisetron) as effective as Zofran (ondansetron) in cisplatin-induced emesis? Anticancer Drugs 6 : 15–21

45. Navari RM, Kaplan HG, Gralla RJ, Grunberg SM, Palmer R, Fitts D (1994) Efficacy and safety of Granisetron, a selective 5-hydroxy-tryptamine-3 receptor antagonist, in the prevention of nausea and vomiting induced by high-dose cisplatin. J Clin Oncol 12 : 2204–2210

46. Navari R, Gandara D, Hesketh P, Hall S, Mailliard J, Ritter H, Friedman C, Fitts D on behalf of the Granisetron Study Group (1995) Comparative clinical trial of granisetron and ondansetron in the prophylaxis of cisplatin-induced emesis. J Clin Oncol 12 : 1242–1245

47. Nicolai N, Mangiarotti B, Salvioni R et al (1993) Dexamethasone plus ondansetron versus dexamethasone plus alizapride in the prevention of emesis induced by cisplatin-containing chemotherapies for urological cancers. Eur Urol 23 : 450–456

48. Palmer R, Moriconi W, Cohn J et al (1995) A double-blind comparison of the efficacy and safety of oral granisetron with oral prochlorperazine in preventing nausea and emesis inpatients receiving moderately emetogenic chemotherapy. Proc Am Soc Clin Oncol 14 : 528 (# 1740)

49. Perez EA, Hesketh PJ, Gandara DR (1991) Serotonin antagonists in the management of cisplatin-induced emesis. Semin Oncol 18 [Suppl 3] : 73–80

50. Perez EA (1995) Review of the preclinical pharmacology and comparative efficacy of 5-hydroxytryptamine-3 receptor antagonists for chemotherapy-induced emesis. J Clin Oncol 13 : 1036–1043

51. Perez EA, Chawla SP, Kaywin PK, Sandbach K, Yocom K, Preston A, Friedman C (1997) Efficacy and safety of oral granisetron versus IV ondansetron in prevention of moderately emetogenic chemotherapy-induced nausea and vomiting. Proc Am Soc Clin Oncol 16 : 43a (#149)

52. Rath U, Upadhyaya BK, Arechavala E et al (1993) Role of ondansetron plus dexamethasone in fractionated chemotherapy. Oncology 50 : 168–172

53. Riviere A, on behalf of the Granisetron Study Group (1994) Dose finding study of granisetron in patients receiving high-dose cisplatin chemotherapy. Br J Cancer 69 : 967–971

54. Roila F, Tonato M, Cognetti F, Cortesi E, Favalli G, Marangolo M, Amadori D, Bella MA, Gramazio V, Donati D, Ballatori E, Del Favero A (1991) Prevention of cisplatin-induced emesis: a double-blind multicenter randomized crossover study comparing ondansetron and ondansetron plus dexamethasone. J Clin Oncol 9 : 675–678

55. Rubenstein EB, Gralla RJ, Hainsworth JD, Hesketh PJ, Grote TH, Modiano MR, Khojasteh A, Kalman LA, Benedict CR, Hahne WF (1997) Randomized, double-blind, dose-response trial across four oral doses of dolasetron for the prevention of acute emesis after moderately emetogenic chemotherapy. Oral Dolasetron Dose-Response Study Group. Cancer 79 : 1216–1224

56. Ruff P, Paska W, Goedhals L, Pouiliart P, Riviere A, Vorolieof D, Bloch, Jones A, Martin, Brunet R, Butcher, Forster J, McQuade B, on behalf of the Ondansetron and Granisetron Emesis Study Group (1994) Ondansetron compared with granisetron in the prophylaxis of cisplatin-induced acute emesis: a multicenter double-blind, randomized, parallel-group study. Oncology 51 : 113–118

57. Seynaeve C, Schuller J, Buser K, Porteder H, Van Belle S, Sevelda P, Christmann D, Schmidt M, Kitchener H, Paes D, de Mulder PHM, on behalf of the Ondansetron Study Group (1992) Comparison of the antiemetic efficacy of ondansetron given as either a continuous infusion or a single intravenous dose, in acute cisplatin-induced emesis. A multicenter, double-blind, randomized, parallel group study. Br J Cancer 66 : 192–197

58. Sledge GW, Einhorn L, Nagy C et al (1992) Phase III double-blind comparison of intravenous ondansetron and metoclopramide as antiemetic therapy for patients receiving multiple-day cisplatin-based chemotherapy. Cancer 70 : 2524–2528

59. Soukop M, McQuade B, Hunter E et al (1992) Ondansetron compared with metoclopramide in the control of emesis and quality of life during repeated chemotherapy for breast cancer. Oncology 49 : 295–304

60. Soukop M, on behalf of the Granisetron Study Group (1994) A dose-finding study of granisetron, a novel antiemetic, in patients receiving high-dose cisplatin. Support Care Cancer 2 : 177–183

61. Tattersall FD, Rycroft W, Hill RG, Hargreaves RJ (1994) Enantioselective inhibition of apomorphine-induced emesis in the ferret by the neurokinin1 receptor antagonist CP-99,994. Neuropharmacocology 33 : 259–260

62. Thant M, Pendergras K, Harman G, Modiano M, Martin L, DuBois D, Cramer M, Hahne W (1996) Double-blind, randomized study of the dose-response relationship across five single doses of IV dolasetron mesylate (DM) for prevention of acute nausea and vomiting (ANC) after cisplatin chemotherapy (CCT). Proc Am Soc Clin Oncol 15 : 533 (#1727)

63. Van Belle SJ-P, Stamatakis L, Bleiberg H, Cocquyt FJ, Michel J, de Bruijn KM (1994) Dose-finding study of tropisetron in cisplatin-induced nausea and vomiting. Ann Oncol 5 : 821–825

64. Warr D, Willan A, Fine S et al (1991) Superiority of granisetron to dexamethasone plus prochlorperazine in the prevention of chemotherapy-induced emesis. J Natl Cancer Inst 83 : 1169–1173

Anticipatory Nausea and Vomiting in the Era of 5-HT$_3$ Antiemetics

Gary R. Morrow, Joseph A. Roscoe, Jeffrey J. Kirshner, Harry E. Hynes, Richard J. Rosenbluth

ABSTRACT Cancer chemotherapy is known to lead to nausea and vomiting in a large proportion of cases. If emesis is severe it can lead in its turn to anticipatory nausea and vomiting (ANV), which cannot be controlled by antiemetic medication. The etiology of ANV and various methods that have been used to counteract the condition are discussed.

Introduction

Patients have reported nausea and vomiting (NV) following the administration of chemotherapy ever since the drugs were first used to treat cancers. Fortunately, since that time, pharmacological control of chemotherapy-induced nausea and emesis has improved. Still, even with the widespread use of the new 5-HT$_3$ antiemetic agents, such as ondansetron, approximately 40% of patients still develop emesis following chemotherapy and over 75% report nausea. If not adequately controlled, these side effects can lead to further complications, such as anorexia and metabolite imbalance, and also contribute to a general deterioration of the cancer patient's psychological and physical condition [4]. The impact of inadequately controlled NV on patient's quality of life is also substantial. One commonly reported consequence, caused by the conditioning effect created by frequent and/or severe post-treatment NV, is the advent of anticipatory NV (ANV). ANV, which develop in approximately 30% of patients by the fourth treatment cycle, appears to link psychological, neurological, and physiological systems [5]. Once they develop, ANV cannot be controlled by antiemetics, including the new 5-HT$_3$ receptor antagonists. Fortunately, behavioral interventions have been effective in mitigating these side effects, and low doses of the anxiolytic agent alprazolam may be potentially useful as a pharmacological preventive intervention [36]. This paper will examine these interventions as well as the prevalence and etiology of ANV.

Etiology

Several characteristics of ANV suggested that its mechanisms might fit within a learning model. Potential conditioned stimuli (such as the sight of the nurse or other sights, sounds, or smells of the clinic) are present while the chemotherapeutic agents (unconditioned stimulus) that produce the unconditioned response (nausea and emesis) are administered. Over several trials (chemotherapy cycles), the conditioned response stimuli (sights, sounds, and even thoughts of the clinic) can be learned; they then produce what is now the conditioned response of ANV. The frequency of ANV increases almost linearly with the number of chemotherapy cycles given [29] and is related to both the frequency [41] and severity of posttreatment NV. Anticipatory side effects seldom develop unless posttreatment side effects have occurred. Few patients in our series of over 4000 developed anticipatory nausea without having experienced posttreatment nausea at least once. Other research also supports the conclusion that ANV involves elements of classical conditioning [3–5, 31, 38–40], and no data convincingly contradict the conclusion that ANV is learned.

Several investigators have speculated that anxiety may be involved in the development of anticipatory side effects. Andrykowski [2] and Andrykowski et al. [3] provided evidence that elevated levels of state anxiety may precede the initial occurrence of anticipatory symptoms. These authors caution, however, that the relationship between anxiety and anticipatory side effects may not be a strictly causal one. Their data also support a view that anxiety may be heightened following a particular chemotherapy treatment and that, in turn, the increased anxiety may increase posttreatment NV which, in turn, may increase susceptibility to conditioning on the next chemotherapy cycle. This circular process may facilitate and promote a conditioning process rather than serve as a direct cause itself. It is likely that some degree of anxiety facilitates the conditioning process by alerting or sensitizing the patient in much the same way as somebody who is mildly anxious may be quite prone to suddenly notice and become concerned over a physical sensation, such as irregular heart beats, that had probably been present for a period of time.

A further complication to fully understanding the relationship between anxiety and ANV is that anxiety, which develops initially as a consequence of chemotherapy-related NV, can itself become a conditioned response [10, 15, 19, 35]. This may lead to a situation in which both ANV and anticipatory anxiety develop as a consequence of repeated nausea-producing chemotherapy treatments [18, 38], with each possibly contributing to the magnitude of the other.

It is also known that autonomic, particularly sympathetic, reactivity correlates with the development of conditioned responses. Kvale's group [20, 21] has demonstrated a connection between autonomic reactivity and subsequent development of ANV. Patients in both studies who experienced ANV showed significantly increased sympathetic reactivity compared with patients who did not experience ANV. Similarly, Challis and Stam [8] found that patients who experienced ANV showed significantly higher levels of awareness concerning their autonomic activity than did patients who did not experience ANV. Another group of investigators found increased parasympathetic autonomic conditionability, measured by the development of conditioned heart rate deceleration, in patients with a history of conditioned nausea in response to chemotherapy; patients without conditioned nausea did not develop the conditioned heart rate deceleration [13]. These findings are suggestive of a mediational role for autonomic reactivity in ANV development.

Prevalence

The average prevalence of ANV compiled from 35 published studies [33] comprising 4382 adult and pediatric cancer chemotherapy patients was 29% for anticipatory nausea and 11% for anticipatory vomiting. Reported rates among the studies varied widely. On the lower end of estimates, 18% of 71 patients examined by Nicholas [34] reported anticipatory side effects, while Cella et al. [7] reported that over half of 60 patients previously treated for Hodgkin's disease developed ANV. Factors that contribute to this variance in rates include differences in: (1) the emetic potential of the chemotherapy drugs administered, (2) measurement methodology (e.g., what treatment cycle was investigated, whether reports were compiled retrospectively or as patient logs, and whether or not NV symptoms were recorded independently of each other or combined as one phenomenon), and (3) the definition of NV (i.e., some investigators record any nausea or vomiting that occurs during chemotherapy treatment as anticipatory effects, whereas other researchers consider NV symptoms at that time to be a physiological response to the chemotherapy drugs).

Perhaps the best way to avoid some of the methodological and definitional issues associated with this field of research is to look primarily at the University of Rochester Cancer Center study. We collected data on 2877 patients treated in geographically diverse member sites of the URCC Community Clinical Oncology Program, all of whom were assessed with the same scale (Morrow Assessment of Nausea and Emesis [26]) at a standard point in their treatment (prior to the fourth chemotherapy cycle). It appears that the cross-sectional prevalence rate for anticipatory nausea is around 20%, with approximately one third of all patients experiencing the symptom at least once by the fourth treatment. Approximately 8% of patients had at least one occurrence of anticipatory vomiting during this time period.

We compared patterns of chemotherapy-related NV in a group of 300 of these patients treated consecutively just prior to the availability of 5-HT$_3$ antiemetics (September 1987 to January 1991) with those of the 300 most recently treated patients (September 1993 to February 1995). Age and gender were comparable between groups. Eighty-six percent of the patients in the later group received 5-HT$_3$ antiemetics. A significant reduction over time in the number of patients reporting at least one episode of posttreatment vomiting (51.7% and 41.3%, $p<0.02$), but no difference in posttreatment nausea (78.7% and 76.7%, $p>0.5$) was found. No significant differences were seen in the reported severity of either symptom. A significant increase in the average duration of both posttreatment nausea (from 28.1 h to 37.2 h, $p<0.002$) and posttreatment vomiting (from 10.8 h to 16.5 h, $p<0.02$) occurred.

The numbers of patients experiencing at least one episode of anticipatory nausea (from 31.0% to 32.0%) or anticipatory vomiting (from 8.3% to 6.3%) were not significantly different ($p>0.3$) for all comparisons. Nor were there significant differences between groups in duration or severity of anticipatory symptoms ($p>0.3$ for all comparisons).

Pharmacological Treatment

Antiemetics do not control ANV once it has developed and indeed have been found by some investigators to paradoxically increase symptoms [6, 23, 25, 28, 30, 32], perhaps by acting as conditioned stimuli themselves [30]. Once developed, ANV does not appear to improve spontaneously [30, 32]. A preliminary study by Razavi et al. [36] does suggest, though, that a potentially useful pharmacological preventive intervention may be low-dose alprazolam (0.5–2 mg) taken daily. Razavi et al.'s double-blind, placebo-controlled study of 57 women with breast cancer found a significantly higher occurrence of anticipatory nausea (18% vs 0%) in the placebo arm than in the alprazolam arm of the study. This significant difference between groups was found prior to the third treatment but not at later treatments.

Behavioral Treatment

Systematic desensitization (SD), or counterconditioning, is a well-developed, standardized behavioral technique that is effective against ANV associated with cancer chemotherapy [11, 14, 16, 24, 28]. A key element of SD is the construction of a hierarchy of events related to the original stimulus that elicit the maladaptive response in each patient. This hierarchy might include events related to administration of chemotherapy, such as driving to the clinic, entering the treatment room, and seeing the clinic nurse. Following this, the patient is trained to associate an alternative response (e.g., deep muscle relaxation) with these events [27, 28]. SD can be taught to patients in about 20 min, and properly trained nurses and oncologists can clinically use SD with about the same effectiveness as can trained behavioral consultants [32].

Hypnosis has been shown in several studies, most of them involving children and adolescents, to be effective in treating ANV [6, 9, 17, 22, 42, 43]. It is a self-control technique in which patients learn to invoke a physiological state incompatible with NV [37]. In the method usually used to produce the altered state of consciousness, induction of total body relaxation is followed by presentation of restful psychic imagery. Suggestions for specific treatment objectives, such as increasing food intake, can then be made [13, 22] or subjects can be led to visualize a series of events (e.g., those associated with ANV), a technique similar to SD [37]. Patients can undergo chemotherapy while hypnotized [37].

Conclusions

Currently available pharmacological agents are still unable to provide complete protection from either anticipatory or posttreatment nausea and emesis associated with chemotherapy. While the introduction of the 5-HT$_3$ antiemetics has led to a reduction in the frequency of posttreatment vomiting, this comes at the apparent expense of an increase in the duration of posttreatment nausea and emesis when they do occur. Therapeutic effects on anticipatory symptomatology have been limited. A multidisciplinary approach that includes the best possible pharmacological control of postchemotherapy NV, drugs as needed to decrease anxiety, and adjunctive behavioral treatment, ideally given prophylactically [1, 12, 22, 23, 25], remains the best treatment option for ANV.

ACKNOWLEDGEMENTS This work was supported by National Cancer Institute grant CA37420.

References

1. Andrews PLR, Sanger GJ (eds) (1993) Emesis in anti-cancer therapy. Mechanisms and treatment. Chapman and Hall Medical, London
2. Andrykowski MA (1990) The role of anxiety in the development of anticipatory nausea in cancer chemotherapy: a review and synthesis (review). Psychosom Med 52 : 458–475
3. Andrykowski MA, Redd WH, Hatfield AK (1985) Development of anticipatory nausea: a prospective analysis. J Consult Clin Psychol 53 : 447–454
4. Bilgrami S, Fallon BG (1993) Chemotherapy-induced nausea and vomiting. Easing patients' fear and discomfort with effective antiemetic regimens (review). Postgrad Med 94 : 55–58
5. Burish TG, Carey MP (1986) Conditioned aversive responses in cancer chemotherapy patients: theoretical and developmental analysis (review). J Consult Clin Psychol 54 : 593–600
6. Carey MP, Burish TG (1988) Etiology and treatment of the psychological side effects associated with cancer chemotherapy: a critical review and discussion (review). Psychol Bull 104 : 307–325
7. Cella DF, Pratt A, Holland JC (1984) Long-term conditioned nausea and anxiety persisting in cured Hodgkin's patients after chemotherapy. Proc Ann Mtg Am Soc Clin Oncol 3 : 73
8. Challis GB, Stam HJ (1992) A longitudinal study of the development of anticipatory nausea and vomiting in cancer chemotherapy patients: the role of absorption and autonomic perception. Health Psychol 11 : 181–189
9. Cotanch P, Hockenberry M, Herman S (1985) Self-hypnosis as antiemetic therapy in children receiving chemotherapy. Oncol Nurs Forum 12 : 41–46
10. DiLorenzo TA, Jacobsen PB, Bovbjerg DH, Chang H, Hudis CA, Sklarin NT, Norton L (1995) Sources of anticipatory emotional distress in women receiving chemotherapy for breast cancer. Ann Oncol 6 : 705–711
11. Elam CL, Andrykowski MA (1991) Admission interview ratings: relationship to applicant academic and demographic variables and interviewer characteristics. Acad Med 66 [Suppl 9] : 13–15
12. Fallowfield LJ (1992) Behavioural interventions and psychological aspects of care during chemotherapy. Eur J Cancer [A] 28 [Suppl 1] : 39–41
13. Fredrikson M, Hursti T, Salmi P, Borjeson S, Furst CJ, Peterson C, Steineck G (1993) Conditioned nausea after cancer chemotherapy and autonomic nervous system conditionability. Scand J Psychol 34 : 318–327
14. Hailey BJ, White JG (1983) Systematic desensitization for anticipatory nausea associated with chemotherapy. Psychosomatics 24 : 287–291
15. Hall JF (1986) The conditional emotional response as a model of Pavlovian conditioning. Pavlovian J Biol Sci 21 : 1–11
16. Hoffman ML (1983) Hypnotic desensitization for the management of anticipatory emesis in chemotherapy. Am J Clin Hypnosis 2 : 173–176
17. Jacknow DS, Tschann JM, Link MP, Boyce WT (1994) Hypnosis in the prevention of chemotherapy-related nausea and vomiting in children: a prospective study. J Dev Behav Pediatrics 15 : 258–264
18. Jacobsen PB, Bovbjerg DH, Redd WH (1993) Anticipatory anxiety in women receiving chemotherapy for breast cancer. Health Psychol 12 : 469–475

19. Jacobsen PB, Bovbjerg DH, Schwartz MD, Hudis CA, Gilewski TA, Norton L (1995) Conditioned emotional distress in women receiving chemotherapy for breast cancer. J Consult Clin Psychol 63 : 108–114

20. Kvale G, Hugdahl K, Asbjornsen A, Rosengren B, Lote K, Nordby H (1991) Anticipatory nausea and vomiting in cancer patients. J Consult Clin Psychol 59 : 894–898

21. Kvale G, Psychol C, Hugdahl K (1994) Cardiovascular conditioning and anticipatory nausea and vomiting in cancer patients. Behav Med 20 : 78–83

22. LaBaw W, Holton C, Tewell K, Eccles D (1975) The use of self-hypnosis by children with cancer. Am J Clin Hypnosis 17 : 233–238

23. Morrow GR (1984) Clinical characteristics associated with the development of anticipatory nausea and vomiting in cancer patients undergoing chemotherapy treatment. J Clin Oncol 2 : 1170–1176

24. Morrow GR (1986) Effect of the cognitive hierarchy in the systematic desensitization treatment of anticipatory nausea in cancer patients: a component comparison with relaxation only, counseling, and no treatment. Cogn Ther Res 10 : 421–446

25. Morrow GR (1989) Chemotherapy-related nausea and vomiting: etiology and management (review). CA Cancer J Clin 39 : 89–104

26. Morrow GR (1992) A patient report measure for the quantification of chemotherapy induced nausea and emesis: psychometric properties of the Morrow assessment of nausea and emesis (MANE). Br J Cancer Suppl 19 : S72–74

27. Morrow GR, Dobkin PL (1988) Anticipatory nausea and vomiting in cancer patients undergoing chemotherapy treatment: prevalence, etiology, and behavioral interventions. Clin Psychol Rev 8 : 517–556

28. Morrow GR, Morrell C (1982) Behavioral treatment for the anticipatory nausea and vomiting induced by cancer chemotherapy. N Engl J Med 307 : 1476–1480

29. Morrow GR, Rosenthal SN (1996) Models, mechanisms and management of anticipatory nausea and emesis (review). Oncology 53 [Suppl 1] : 4–7

30. Morrow GR, Arseneau JC, Asbury RF, Bennett JM, Boros L (1982) Anticipatory nausea and vomiting with chemotherapy. N Engl J Med 306 : 431–432

31. Morrow GR, Lindke J, Black PM (1991) Predicting development of anticipatory nausea in cancer patients: prospective examination of eight clinical characteristics. J Pain Symptom Manage 6 : 215–223

32. Morrow GR, Asbury R, Hammon S, Dobkin P, Caruso L, Pandya K, Rosenthal S (1992) Comparing the effectiveness of behavioral treatment for chemotherapy-induced nausea and vomiting when administered by oncologists, oncology nurses and clinical psychologists. Health Psychol 11 : 250–256

33. Morrow GR, Roscoe JA, Hickok JT (1998) Treatment induced nausea and vomiting: etiology and management. In: Holland JC (ed) Handbook of psychooncology (in press)

34. Nicholas DR (1982) Prevalence of anticipatory nausea and emesis in cancer chemotherapy patients. J Behav Med 5 : 461–463

35. Rachman S (1991) Neo-conditioning and the classical theory of fear acquisition. Clin Psychol Rev 11 : 155–173

36. Razavi D, Delvaux N, Farvacques C, De Brier F, Van Heer C, Kaufman L, Derde M-P, Piccart M (1993) Prevention of adjustment disorders and anticipatory nausea secondary to adjuvant chemotherapy: a double-blind, placebo-controlled study assessing the usefulness of alprazolam. J Clin Oncol 11 : 1384–1390

37. Redd WH, Andresen GV, Minagawa RY (1982) Hypnotic control of anticipatory emesis in patients receiving cancer chemotherapy. J Consult Clin Psychol 50 : 14–19

38. Sabbioni ME, Bovbjerg DH, Jacobsen PB, Manne SL, Redd WH (1992) Treatment related psychological distress during adjuvant chemotherapy as a conditioned response. Ann Oncol 3 : 393–398

39. Schwartz MD, Jacobsen PB, Bovbjerg DH (1996) Role of nausea in the development of aversions to a beverage paired with chemotherapy treatment in cancer patients. Physiol Behav 59 : 659–663

40. Stockhorst U, Klosterhalfen S, Klosterhalfen W, Winkelmann M, Steingrueber HJ (1993) Anticipatory nausea in cancer patients receiving chemotherapy: classical conditioning etiology and therapeutical implications. Integrative Physiol Behav Sci 28 : 177–181

41. Tomoyasu N, Bovbjerg DH, Jacobsen PB (1996) Conditioned reactions to cancer chemotherapy: percent reinforcement predicts anticipatory nausea. Physiol Behav 2 : 273–276

42. Zeltzer L, LeBaron S (1982) Hypnosis and nonhypnotic techniques for reduction of pain and anxiety during painful procedures in children and adolescents with cancer. Behav Pediatr 101 : 1032–1035

43. Zeltzer LK, Dolgin MJ, LeBaron S, LeBaron C (1991) A randomized, controlled study of behavioral intervention for chemotherapy distress in children with cancer. Pediatrics 88 : 34–42

Consensus Regarding Multiple-Day and Rescue Antiemetic Therapy

Pieter H. M. De Mulder, Fausto Roila, Mark G. Kris, Michel M. Marty

ABSTRACT Different forms of moderately and highly emetogenic cancer chemotherapy that are administered over several days per cycle are discussed with reference to the most efficacious antiemetic therapy. Both preventive and rescue antiemetic therapy are considered.

Multiple-Day Chemotherapy

A considerable number of chemotherapeutic regimens are given over more than 1 day. Most of these combinations comprise both moderately and highly emetogenic agents. To date no studies have evaluated the use of antiemetics in the prevention of mildly emetogenic chemotherapy administered over multiple days and therefore none can be included in this review.

The most commonly used combination fulfilling this criterion is 5-day low-dose cisplatin given mostly in combination with etoposide/ifosfamide and bleomycin. This is the treatment of choice for metastatic germ cell tumors and undifferentiated tumors of unknown origin. This patient category comprises mainly younger patients, who are especially susceptible for the extrapyramidal side effects associated with the use of high-dose metoclopramide.

With the recognition of the importance of the 5-HT_3 receptors in the mediation of acute chemotherapy-induced nausea and vomiting (NV), setrons became the first drugs of choice. The pathophysiology of NV when emetogenic chemotherapy is given over more than 1 day is complicated by the fact that after 1 day both the "acute" and the "delayed" pathway are stimulated. The 5-HT_3 receptor plays a predominant role in acute NV, while the predominant receptor(s) in the delayed phase are ill defined. The pattern of emesis observed over 5 days of cisplatin with prochlorperazine [11] reveals a peak on day 1 with a steep decline thereafter. This indicates that on the second day a similar dose of cisplatin elicits a lower stimulus or that the stimuli causing delayed emesis are more dominant, thus suppressing the acute pathway. There is of course no formal proof for this supposition, but it might explain what has been observed. The early phase II data with 5-HT$_3$ antagonists show a pattern that may further support this hypothesis. The highest level of protection is seen on day 1 (75%) [9, 10], with a clear loss of efficacy thereafter despite continuation of the same treatment. The existence of this pattern is relevant to review the results obtained so far with antiemetic therapy over multiple-day cisplatin treatment.

In three randomized studies, 5-HT$_3$ antagonists were shown to be superior (30–50% complete protection over 5 days) to metoclopramide, alizapride with dexamethasone, and metoclopramide combined with dexamethasone. In one of the first published double-blind, randomized studies, ondansetron three times daily (0.15 mg/kg q 4 h) was compared with metoclopramide (1 mg/kg three times daily with a similar time interval) [17]. In this relatively small study 45 patients were entered. The failure rate, defined as more than five emetic episodes during a 24-h period, was significantly less with ondansetron, at 9% versus 50% for the metoclopramide-treated patients (p=0.002). There were seven patients treated with ondansetron who experienced no vomiting over the whole 5-day period, compared with two treated with metoclopramide (p=0.077). An analysis per day indicated the largest difference in efficacy on day 1 (78% versus 14%). As might be expected, the incidence of extrapyramidal side effects was significantly higher in the metoclopramide-treated group. It is of course relevant that total protection in the ondansetron-treated patients over the whole period was relatively poor, with 70% of the patients experiencing at least one emetic period. The pattern of control observed in this study was similar to that observed in the previous phase II studies. In contrast, patients treated with metoclopramide showed an inverse pattern, with the highest reported protection on day 5 (50% on day 5 versus 14% on day 1). In view of these results, together with the significantly better toxicity profile, 5-HT$_3$ antagonist are the drugs of choice. Although no formal studies have been done with the now established optimal lowest dose of the various setrons, there are no compelling arguments for not recommending these doses for the multiple-day indication (ondansetron 8 mg i.v., granisetron 1 mg i.v., and tropisetron 5 mg i.v., all given once daily prior to the start of chemotherapy).

To improve on these results, the logic next step was the combination of setrons with corticosteroids (dexamethasone or methylprednisolone). This issue has been addressed in three randomized studies, and a significant therapeutic advantage has been shown for the addition of corticosteroids. The combination of a 5-HT$_3$ receptor antagonist plus dexamethasone has been shown to induce about 55–83% of complete protection from vomiting during the 3–5 days of cisplatin administration, and this combination has been shown to be superior to high-dose metoclopramide plus dexamethasone [17], to alizapride plus dexamethasone [16], and to ondansetron alone

[15]. In the study by Fox et al. [8], ondansetron was combined with both chlorpromazine (a dopamine antagonist) and dexamethasone. In this open-label study with 44 patients treated with either ondansetron (0.15 mg/kg × 3 for 4 or 5 days) or ondansetron plus 2 days dexamethasone (8 mg at –30 min, followed by 4 mg × 2 every 4 h) and oral chlorpromazine (50 mg every 4 h × 4 for 4 or 5 days), there was no difference in complete control for the whole 5-day period, but 86% of the patients treated with the triple combination experienced only three emetic episodes over 5 days, versus 46% for ondansetron alone. In view of the low number of patients treated, this study lacks the power to detect even meaningful differences in complete control, but the trend is clear. The contribution of chlorpromazine in this study cannot be separated from that of dexamethasone, and its relative value is therefore unclear. The use of this compound does have a rationale, in view of the earlier mentioned potential role in the delayed pathway. This study with the low number of patients is not sufficient to allow any conclusion, but the trends it shows up could be investigated further.

In another double-blind parallel-group study, 32 mg ondansetron bolus plus 20 mg dexamethasone was compared with metoclopramide alone (2 or 1 mg/kg at –30 min and +90 min) and plus the same dexamethasone dose [16]. No preventive measures were taken to avoid extrapyramidal side effects. In the combination arm, 71% experienced two emetic episodes or fewer over the whole 5-day period, versus 26% for the metoclopramide alone arm.

With 40 µg/kg granisetron, 54% complete protection over 5 days has been observed in a single-blind randomized study with 200 patients. Within the control arm, whose patients were receiving 4 mg/kg alizapride followed by 4 mg/kg 2 × every 4 h plus 8 mg dexamethasone, there was 43% complete control. The difference was not significant. Only on day 1 was there a significant difference in favor of granisetron (90% versus 65.9%, $p>0.001$) [2].

Little is known about the optimal dose and timing of corticosteroids in this context. For patients treated with curative intent, one should realize that, although rare, serious side effects (such as aseptic necrosis of bone of mainly head of femur and cataract) have been described after high-dose corticosteroids. In 5-day cisplatin regimens corticosteroids are given for 5 consecutive days every 3 weeks for a total of 12 weeks, repeated to give four cycles in all. The side effects of 5-HT$_3$ anatagonists are low and reversible.

Other regimens given over 5 days or longer include oral CMF. This is a very frequently used multiple-day regimen with oral cyclophosphamide given over 14 days. Two studies address this problem. In the study by Buser [3], ondansetron over the whole 14-day period was superior to placebo. In a second study [13], ondansetron was equally effective in the control of emesis as the combination dexamethasone i.v. on days 1 and 8 plus 3 × 10 mg oral metoclopramide every day during oral cyclophosphamide treatment, but nausea was better controlled on days 1 and 2 with the latter combination. A total of 164 patients were included in this study. There is no other study available to confirm this observation. Is this the final answer? The value of the 3×10 mg oral metoclopramide is limited, but it might be enough to protect against the emetogenic potential of oral cyclophosphamide.

Dacarbazine is a highly emetogenic drug; in fact, all patients treated with 250 mg/m^2 daily for 5 days suffered from NV.

Based on a pilot study demonstrating that high-dose metoclopramide prevents emesis in four out of ten patients [18], a randomized double-blind study comparing high-dose metoclopramide alone (2 mg/kg i.v. $\times$ 4 for 2 days) versus metoclopramide (at the same dose and schedule) combined with methylprednisolone (250 mg i.v. twice daily for 2 days) has been carried out in 34 patients treated with 250 mg/m^2 dacarbazine daily for 5 days [1]. On day 1 there was no difference in efficacy between the two antiemetic regimens (66% of patients had complete protection from vomiting), but on day 2 metoclopramide plus methylprednisolone was significantly superior to metoclopramide alone (100% vs 71%). Interestingly, after antiemetic therapy was stopped, nearly one third of patients experienced emesis.

The activity of the 5-HT$_3$ receptor antagonists in combination with steroids has not been compared with that of a combination of metoclopramide plus steroids in dacarbazine-treated patients. Today it would be difficult to carry out such a study, since it has been demonstrated that in cisplatin-treated patients the 5-HT$_3$ receptor antagonist plus steroid combination is superior to high-dose metoclopramide combinations [12].

The optimal duration of antiemetic therapy should be determined in patients treated with fractionated dacarbazine.

Consensus for the Control of Emesis Caused by Chemotherapy Given over Multiple Days

1. The optimal antiemetic regimen, based on the emetogenic potential of the chemotherapeutic agents, should be repeated on each day of therapy.
   Level of scientific confidence: High
   Level of consensus: High

2. For control of emesis during cisplatin treatment, a 5-HT$_3$ receptor antagonist plus dexamethasone given on each day is the treatment of choice.
   Level of scientific confidence: High
   Level of consensus: Moderate for patients treated with curative intent,
   high for palliative intent

3. For dacarbazine, a 5-HT$_3$ receptor antagonist plus dexamethasone given
   on each day of chemotherapy is the treatment of choice.
   Level of scientific confidence: Very low
   Level of consensus: High

4. With the present recommended combination for multiple-day cisplatin
   treatment, the level of complete control declines on successive days compared with the first day of treatment. Further studies are needed.
   Level of scientific confidence: High
   Level of consensus: High

5. With oral CMF, dexamethasone on day 1 and 8 in combination with
   14 days' oral metoclopramide is the treatment of choice. A 5-HT$_3$ antagonist should be used only when the above-mentioned combination is not
   tolerated.
   Level of scientific confidence: Moderate
   Level of consensus: Moderate

6. More studies should be carried out in patients undergoing multiple days of
   moderately emetogenic therapy (i.e., ifosfamide) or mildly emetogenic
   chemotherapy (i.e., fluorouracil).
   Level of scientific confidence: Not applicable
   Level of consensus: High

Rescue Medication

Rescue medication is required when treatment failure is observed. The definition of failure is the presence of any vomiting and/or moderate to severe
nausea after chemotherapy, providing any form of antiemetic therapy has
been given. The following situations can be discerned: (1) failure during the
first 24 h requiring acute intervention; (2) selection of an alternative for subsequent courses, or decision to give the same regimen once more; (3) failure
in the delayed phase. The definition of failure is given above and applies to all
patients in whom no complete protection against vomiting is seen and those
with more than mild nausea. In daily practice, individual patients may accept
the occurrence of a single episode of vomiting or even two, especially when
there is no moderate to severe nausea over a prolonged period of time. The
subjective evaluation of the patient should be regarded when considering the
limited possibilities for treating a failure. This failure can be observed after
either maximum antiemetic treatment, i.e., optimal-dose 5-HT$_3$ antagonist in
combination with a sufficient dose of corticosteroids (at least 20 mg dexamethasone per day), or after suboptimal treatment or the use of non-5-HT$_3$
antagonists. The latter situation is simple, because there are sufficient data

that indicate that rescue can be obtained by using 5-HT_3 antagonists. Suboptimal treatment means either an insufficient dose of a 5-HT_3 antagonist or this compound alone without corticosteroids. The response to this situation is clear and quite often used in the case of a failure observed when moderately emetogenic cytotoxic agents are used and prophylaxis is given with monotherapy.

The most disturbing clinical situation is that of a failure after optimal treatment. Can a higher dose of the 5-HT_3 antagonists be used? Can another setrons be used? Can a higher or repeated dose of corticosteroids be used? Does the addition of sedatives, such as lorazepam, have a proven value? We all have individual observations on the efficacy of each of the proposed suggestions, but we do not have sound data to support them and to justify extending any of these to a standard approach; clearly more, and obviously difficult, research is required in this area.

In a recent study, rescue therapy was standardized in such a way that a second dose of the same 5-HT_3 antagonist was recommended [14]. Twenty-three patients who originally failed responded to this second dose of the same agent. In five patients, metoclopramide plus dexamethasone in addition to the additional dose of the serotonin antagonist was given. Crossover data in the same study, based on a failure in the previous cycle, provided information on 19 patients. In two complete protection was seen, and in six a major response was seen in the subsequent cycle. This is of course not comparable with a rescue situation, but may suggest an individual variation in sensitivity towards the various setrons. In a phase II setting, patients failing (35 vomits/24 h and/or more than 4 h nausea/24 h) on 5 mg tropisetron i.v. prior to the start of cisplatin were treated with 8 mg ondansetron in the subsequent cycle [4]. In two out of 12, complete protection was found on day 1. In a more recent paper dealing with a larger number of patients, 5 mg tropisetron i.v was given to patients failing previous antiemetic therapy [7]. Failure on previous 5-HT_3 antagonists was defined as more than four nausea/vomiting episodes. In 32% (27/85) complete control was observed in the first tropisetron cycle and 43% control in cycles 2–10, with of course a gradually decreasing number of patients. These data should be considered as anecdotal in view of the design of the studies and may just be the result of chance or intraindividual variance; they are not a scientific basis for advocating crossover from one agent to the other. Addition of drugs with another mechanism of action is more appropriate. In a recent abstract, this approach has been described with the use of metopimazine [5]. A total of 338 patients who experienced at least one emetic episode or nausea during their first course, despite the combination of a 5-HT_3 antagonist with corticosteroids, were randomized in double-blind fashion between ondansetron with methylprednisolone plus or minus metopimazine. Complete control of vomiting was observed in 53% of the patients receiving the triple combination versus 38% for the other arm ($p=0.008$). For nausea a similar pattern was seen ($p=0.03$).

Studies to address the question of failure are complicated in design and require a large number of patients. The following methodological elements should be regarded. The design must be double blind and placebo controlled. The length of follow-up after rescue medication has been given is important. Is 24 h after the start of the chemotherapy long enough? Is a vomit immediately after the start of rescue medication a failure on rescue? If failure occurs during the previous cycle, a uniform definition of failure should be used, and patients should of course have received optimal treatment during the first cycle.

Another attempt to improve control might be the addition of sedatives. Lorazepam is the drug that has most frequently been used in this way, especially in the pre-setron era. In a recent paper describing a study in which cisplatin was administered during sleep [6], prophylactic antiemetic treatment consisted of dexamethasone and ondansetron. In a phase I-like setting, antiemetic treatment was reduced in various steps in those patients who slept. It was possible to reduce the dose of both dexamethasone and ondansetron with more than 80% experiencing no loss of protective efficacy. Although the numbers are low, this observation points to the additional value of sleep, i.e., sedation. With the use of continuous-infusion phenergan and chlorpromazine, which we use as a last step for inpatient rescue, acceptable control can be achieved when the patients are sedated to a level comparable with sleep, but easily arousable (unpublished observations).

Proposed Consensus

1. If optimal treatment has been given as prophylaxis, repeated dosing of the same agents is unlikely to be successful. Administration of a rescue agent or agents of a different pharmacologic class should be attempted.
   Level of scientific confidence: Not applicable
   Level of consensus: High

2. In patients being treated with cisplatin who experience emesis despite optimal antiemetic prophylaxis of acute emesis with a 5-HT_3 antagonist plus dexamethasone, the addition of metopimazine to the antiemetic combination during the following cycle significantly increases the complete protection of acute vomiting and, to a lesser extent, nausea.
   Level of scientific confidence: Low
   Level of consensus: Moderate

3. When vomiting occurs after adequate prophylaxis, other causes of emesis should be considered, such as concomitant medications, bowel obstruction, or brain metastases.

    Level of scientific confidence: Not applicable
    Level of consensus: High

References

1. Basurto C, Roila F, Tonato M et al (1989) Antiemetic activity of high-dose metoclopramide combined with methylprednisolone versus metoclopramide alone in dacarbazine-treated cancer patients. Am J Clin Oncol 12 : 235–238
2. Bremer K on behalf of the granisetron study group (1992) A single-blind study of the efficacy and safety of intravenous granisetron compared with alizapride plus dexamethasone in the prophylaxis and control of emesis in patients receiving 5-day cytostatic therapy. Eur J Cancer [A] 28 : 1018–1022
3. Buser KS, Joss RA, Piquet D et al (1993) Oral ondansetron in the prophylaxis of nausea and vomiting induced by cyclophosphamide, methotrexate and 5-fluorouracil (CMF) in women with breast cancer. Results of a prospective, randomized, double-blind placebocontrolled study. Ann Oncol 4 : 474–479
4. deBoer M, deWit R, Stoter G, Verweij J (1995) Possible lack of full cross-resistance of $5HT_3$ antagonists: a pilot study. Cancer Res Clin Oncol 121 : 126–127
5. Depierre A, Lebeau B, Chevallier B et al (1996) Efficay of ondansetron, methylprednisolone plus metopimazine in patients previously incontrolled with dual therapy in cisplatin containing chemotherapy (abstract). Ann Oncol 7 : 134
6. Domínguez-Ortega L, Cubedo-Cervera R, Cortés-Funés H, Díaz-Gállego E (1996) Sleep protects against chemotherapy induces emesis. Cancer 77 : 1566–1570
7. Falkson C, Falkson H (1995) Antiemetic efficacy of tropisetron in patients failing previous antiemetic therapy. Oncology 52 : 427–431
8. Fox SM, Einhorn LH, Cox E et al (1993) Ondansetron versus ondansetron, dexamethasone, and chlorpromazine in the prevention of nausea and vomiting associated with multiple-day cisplatin chemotherapy. J Clin Oncol 11 : 2391–2395
9. Einhorn LH, Naggy C, Werner K et al (1990) Ondansetron: a new antiemetic for patients receiving cisplatin chemotherapy. J Clin Oncol 8 : 731–735
10. Hainsworth JD (1992) The use of ondansetron in patients receiving multiple-day cisplatin regimens. Semin Oncol 19 : 48–52
11. Herman TS, Einhorn LH, Jones SE et al (1979) Superiority of nabilone over prochlorperazine as an antiemetic in patients receiving cancer chemotherapy. N Engl J Med 300 : 1295–1297
12. Italian Group for Antiemetic Research (1992) Ondansetron + dexamethasone versus metoclopramide + dexamethasone + diphenhydramine in prevention of cisplatin induced emesis. Lancet 340 : 96–99
13. Levitt M, Warr D, Yelle L et al (1993) Ondansetron compared with dexamethasone and metoclopramide as antiemetics in the chemotherapy of breast cancer with cyclophosphamide, methotrexate and fluorouracil. N Engl J Med 328 : 1081–1084
14. Mantovani G, Macciò A, Alessandro B, Curelli L, Ghiani M, Proto E (1996) Comparison of granisetron versus ondansetron versus tropisetron in the prophylaxis of acute nausea and vomiting induced by cisplatin for the treatment of head and neck cancer: a randomized controlled trial. Cancer 77 : 941–948

15. Nicolai N, Mangiarotti B, Salvioni R et al (1993) Dexamethasone plus ondansetron versus dexamethasone plus alizapride in the prevention of emesis induce by cisplatin-containing chemotherapies for urological cancers. Eur Urol 23 : 450–456
16. Räth U, Upadhyaya BK, Arechavala E, et al (1993) Role of ondansetron plus dexamethasone in fractionated chemotherapy. Oncology 50 : 168–172
17. Sledge GW, Einhorn LH, Nagy C et al (1992) Phase III double-blind comparison of intravenous ondansetron and metoclopramide as antiemetic therapy for patients receiving multiple-day cisplatin-based chemotherapy. Cancer 70 : 2524–2528
18. Tyson LB, Clark RA, Gralla RJ (1982) High dose metoclopramide: control of dacarbazine-induced emesis in a preliminary trial. Cancer Treat Rep 66 : 2108

Etiology and Prevention of Emesis Induced by Radiotherapy

Petra C. Feyer, Alan L. Stewart, Otto J. Titlbach

ABSTRACT The introduction of new antiemetics has resulted in renewed interest in the etiology and control of radiation-induced emesis. Studies both with fractionated treatment and with high-dose single exposures have clearly demonstrated the value of the $5\text{-}HT_3$ receptor antagonist antiemetics. This paper reviews the selection of optimal antiemetics.

Introduction

Surgery, radiotherapy, and chemotherapy are the main modalities of cancer treatment. Radiotherapy and surgery are essentially local treatments, in contrast to chemotherapy, and are only curative for local disease.

The therapeutic benefit must take into consideration the degree of tolerable side effects. In the case of curable modalities, a slight increase in side effects is acceptable, but in palliative treatment no reduction in quality of life should be caused by the treatment. Gastrointestinal side effects can complicate curative or palliative radiotherapy, and studies have shown that nausea and vomiting are the most distressing side effects for the patient, producing an adverse effect on quality of life [9].

When radiotherapy is delivered with curative intent, it is essential to have as few breaks in the treatment as possible, since prolonging treatment time may adversely affect tumor control [15, 38]. Effective control of radiation-induced side effects is necessary in order to complete treatment without interruptions. Untreated, emesis persisting through radiotherapy can cause physiologic changes, i.e., dehydration, electrolyte imbalance, and malnutrition, which in turn can hamper the quality of life and the final outcome of treatment [23].

There are important differences between chemotherapy- and radiotherapy-induced emesis, but in general terms nausea and vomiting from radiotherapy is less severe than that seen with more aggressive chemotherapy regimens [32].

The pattern of emesis is easier to determine with single-fraction radiotherapy studies. Radiation has toxic effects similar to those of cytotoxic drugs, but there are fundamental differences in the nature, mechanisms, and actions of chemotherapy and radiation therapy.

The prodromal symptoms (nausea, vomiting, anorexia, and malaise) seen after exposure to radiation are part of a cascade of effects set in motion by the radiation exposure. The latent period prior to the onset of vomiting following irradiation is shorter than that in patients treated with chemotherapy [22]. The pattern of emesis is easier to determine with single-fraction radiotherapy than with fractionated treatment. It is important to understand that during fractionated irradiation the distress to the patient may be particularly pronounced, since the treatment can comprise up to 40 sessions given over a period of 6–8 weeks. The potential for distress to the patient from sickness continuing for that length of time is therefore considerable [37].

Acute emesis is seen most frequently with radiotherapy. The latent period ranges from 30 min to 4 h and, in single-fraction studies, is shorter with higher doses of radiation. Prolonged emesis lasting 2–3 days is reported by up to 40% of patients. Delayed emesis of the pattern seen with cisplatin is not seen with radiotherapy, and anticipatory emesis is extremely rare. Total-body irradiation and irradiation of the upper part of the abdomen or whole abdomen are the most emetogenic radiotherapy regimens and are associated with nausea, vomiting, anorexia, and diarrhea.

Emesis can occur 2–3 weeks after the onset of treatment in approximately 50% of patients receiving conventionally fractionated radiation (1.8–2.0 Gy) to the upper abdomen. Previous reports have indicated that emesis occurs in approximately 50% of patients receiving fractionated radiotherapy to the whole abdomen [33] and in over 80% when single treatments are given [10]. During irradiation of the pelvic region, nausea and emesis are not a frequent clinical problem [28]. An analysis of the management of nausea and vomiting in patients receiving fractionated radiotherapy between thorax and pelvis who were perceived to have a mild to moderate risk for emesis was reported. The analysis included 1387 patients from 11 radiotherapy centers in five countries and showed that approximately 40% of the patients with no antiemetic prophylaxis experienced emesis or nausea [12]. It is clear from this observational study that more attention needs to be given to the selection of patients requiring antiemetic therapy.

Etiology of Radiation-Induced Emesis

The mechanism of emesis after irradiation is complex and multifactorial, being controlled by different factors, including physical as well as physio-

Table 1 Ionizing radiation: emetic sensitivity, latency, and LD_{50} (*latency* time to first emetic episode, ED_{50} dose of radiation required to cause emesis in 50% of the subject population, LD_{50} dose of radiation required to kill 50% of the subject population; in humans, the value is reported as a $LD_{50/60}$, the dose calculated to kill 50% of the subjects within 60 days [19])

Latency	60–90 min
ED_{10}	< 1.0 Gy
ED_{50}	2.0 Gy
ED_{100}	4.0 Gy (ED_{80})
LD_{50}	2.9 Gy

logical and psychological variables. The precise pathophysiology remains unclear.

The pattern of symptoms following a single high dose of irradiation was first described by Court-Brown in 1953 [8]. The pattern consisted of three phases including a latent period, a period of acute disturbances, and a recovery phase. Danjoux et al. [10] described symptoms following hemibody irradiation. The incidence of radiation-induced emesis following hemibody irradiation was higher after mid- and upper hemibody irradiation. These observations made by Court-Brown [8] and Danjoux et al. [10] suggested that the critical organs responsible for radiation-induced emesis were in the upper abdomen and the underlying mechanism might be related to a toxin released by degradation of tumor proteins. The production of a second messenger resulting from radiation-associated cellular damage was also considered. In man, there is no ED_{100} for radiation-induced vomiting (Table 1). Even with the most emetogenic radiotherapy, only 80–90% of patients can be expected to vomit in the absence of antiemetic therapy [2].

Davis et al. [11] have described vomiting in terms of a hierarchically organized toxin defense system in which the irradiated individual responds in a stereotypical manner to a perceived toxin and in this way attempts to protect him- or herself from damage from the toxin. Using this model, vomiting becomes an important postirradiation syndrome.

Experience obtained from the accidents at Tchernobyl in the USSR in 1986 [1] demonstrate that the latency before the onset of emesis is in inverse correlation to the dose (Figs. 1, 2). Hypothetically, there can be two different pathophysiological mechanisms working together in the induction of emesis:
1. Passive cell damage mechanism (histopathological effect) in terms of release of transmitters that induce or contain emesis
2. Active functional defense mechanism (pathophysiological effect) through release of mediators by functioning cells

Free radicals are released immediately after irradiation of cellular tissue. Buell and Harding [6] described an irradiation-induced inflammatory reac-

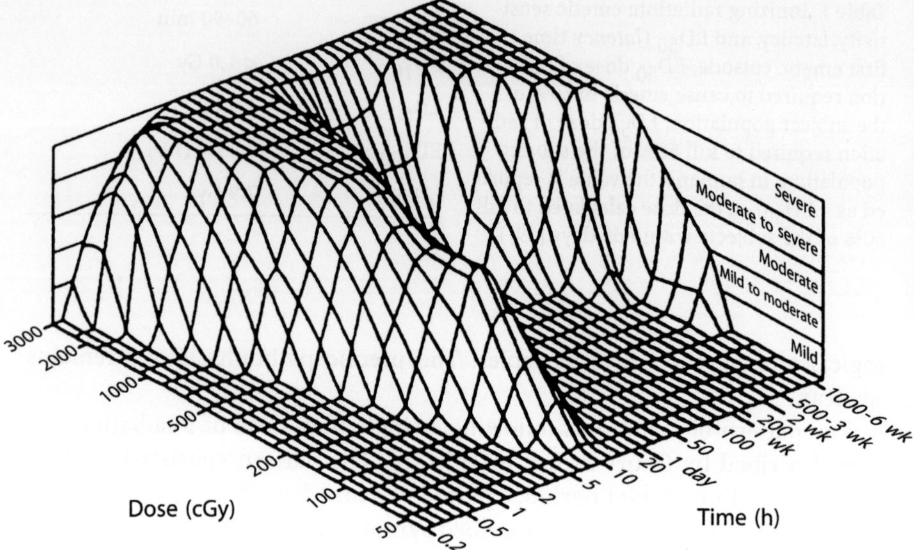

Fig. 1 3-D plot of the relationships between radiation dose, time, and severity of 'upper gastrointestinal symptoms'. Developed from [1, 22]

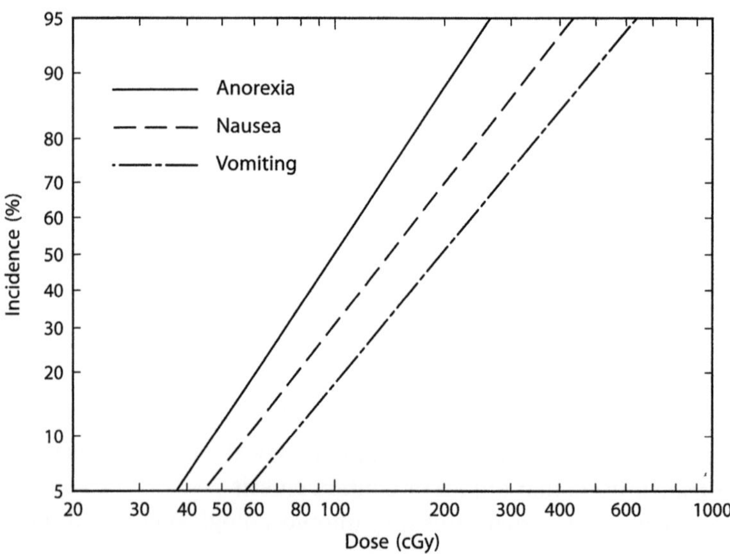

Fig. 2 Relationship of prodromal symptoms (incidence of anorexia, nausea, and vomiting) and radiation dose. (From [22])

tion involving the accumulation of neutrophils in the rat intestinal mucosa immediately after exposure to 10 Gy. These and other data [20, 21] are consistent with a postirradiation inflammatory response. Secondary to the inflammatory reaction there may be release of histamines and other transmitters inducing emesis.

The enterochromaffin cells of the gastrointestinal mucosa have a high serotonin (5-hydroxytryptamine, $5\text{-}HT_3$) content [4]. Damage of the enterochromaffin cells by toxins and/or irradiation leads to release of serotonin, which may initiate the emetogenic response. Serotonin ($5\text{-}HT_3$) may mediate emesis through mechanisms involving $5\text{-}HT_3$ receptors and activation of the chemoreceptor trigger zone (CTZ) in the brain through visceral afferent pathways. The correlation of radiation-induced emesis and levels of 5-hydroxyindoleacetic acid (5-HIAA), a metabolite of $5\text{-}HT_3$, strongly suggests that the mechanism of radiation-induced emesis is related to the release of serotonin. The increase in 5-HIAA after upper and mid-hemibody irradiation and the fact that serotonin is found in high concentrations in the upper abdomen support a model for radiation-induced emesis in which serotonin stimulates the afferent fibers and the CTZ, resulting in emesis [40].

Factors that Influence the Risk of Emesis

Although not all patients experience emesis following radiotherapy, the majority of patients experience it following upper abdominal and total-body irradiation. The frequency, severity, and onset of radiation-induced emesis are related both to the emetogenic potential of the therapy and to the emetogenic risk profile of the patient (Fig. 3). Age, gender, alcohol consumption, and previous experience of emesis are recognized risk factors for emetogenic therapies. Bremer [5] established a score based on the following factors. The risk of emesis is high in female patients, those younger than 50 years, and

Fig. 3 Factors influencing nausea and vomiting

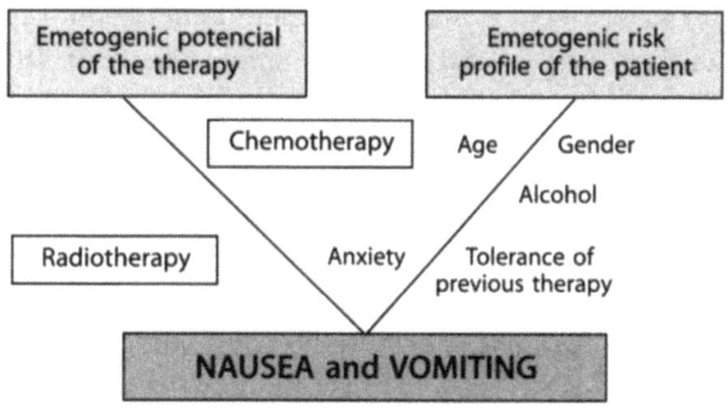

Table 2 Definition of individual risk of emesis with reference to prognostic factors (individual score: ≤5 normal individual emetogenic risk, ≥6 high individual emetogenic risk; Bremer's modification [5])

Emesis risk factor	Score
Age	
> 50 years	1
< 50 years	2
Sex	
Male	1
Female	2
Alcohol consumption	
Yes	1
No	2
Experience of nausea and emesis	
No	1
Yes	2

patients who have a previous history of poorly controlled emesis. Conversely, the risk is decreased in those with a high alcohol intake. Using these factors, an individual risk score can be determined for every patient (Table 2).

Emesis occurs more frequently when patients receive treatment to larger fields [e.g., total-body irradiation (TBI) or hemibody irradiation (HBI)] and in doses higher than 5 Gy. In patients receiving TBI, vomiting has been reported in more than 80% of patients even after premedication with antiemetics [44, 48]. A study reported by Danjoux et al. [10] showed that despite prophylactic non-5-HT$_3$ receptor antagonist antiemetics, radiation-induced emesis occurred within 60 min of treatment in 83% of patients receiving upper HBI and in 30% receiving lower HBI. The difference in the incidence of emesis following upper HBI (> 80%) and lower HBI (30–40%) suggests that the primary organ responsible for the emetic response is in the upper abdomen (Fig. 4).

There can be confusion over the terms "lower" and "upper" HBI. There can be some overlap which influences emetogenic risk. Lower hemibody radiotherapy may extend up to the upper border of the L1 vertebra, thus treating the upper abdomen. Upper hemibody radiotherapy in some centers will extend down to the umbilicus, again irradiating the upper abdominal contents. When reporting results, authors must clearly state the extent of radiation fields used to avoid confusion.

Finally, the most important factors influencing radiation-induced emesis are summarized in Table 3.

Table 3 Factors influencing radiation-induced emesis

- Single and total dose, dose rate
- Fractionation
- Field size
- Irradiated volume
- Site of irradiation
- Organs included in the radiation field
- Patient positioning
- Radiation technique
- Energy, beam quality
- Previous or simultaneous influencing therapy
- General health status of the patient

Fig. 4 Emetogenic potential of radiotherapy site

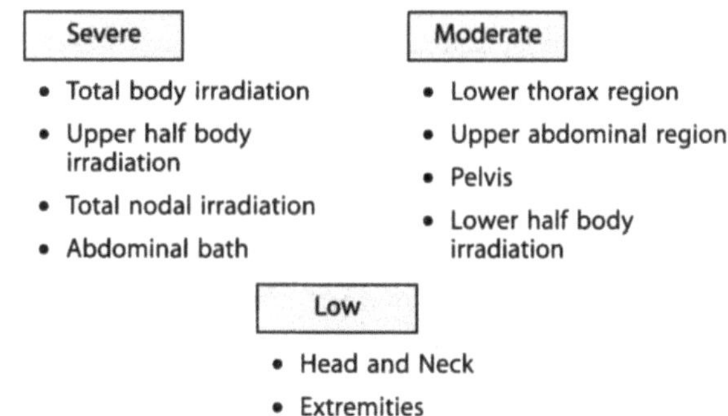

Strategies to Reduce Radiation-Induced Emesis

Primary Prevention

Whenever possible, the risk of emesis should be reduced by modification of the relevant physical factors. When planning treatment, innovative radiotherapy techniques such as 3-D treatment planning, multileaf collimators, and dose volume histograms may reduce the irradiated volume [14].

Chronobiological effects may also be relevant. A recent study by Gagnon and Kuettel [17] has demonstrated that the gastrointestinal tract is more sensitive to radiation-induced damage in the late morning than in the afternoon.

Secondary Prevention

Secondary prevention implies the assessment of emetogenic risk and the use of optimal antiemetic therapy either as prophylaxis prior to radiation or as rescue therapy for established vomiting.

The commonest antiemetics used for prevention of radiation-induced emesis are the benzamides, e.g., metoclopramide or alizapride. They may be used alone or in combination with a neuroleptic, e.g., haloperidol, or a benzodiazepine, e.g., lorazepam or diazepam. The use of 5-HT$_3$ antagonists alone or with a glucocorticoid is usually restricted to the highly emetogenic regimens, e.g., TBI. There are some studies of dopamine antagonists (butyrophenones) in radiotherapy [36] and also of opiate receptor antagonists (cannabinoids) [29, 33].

The Role of 5-HT$_3$ Receptor Antagonists in Radiation-Induced Emesis

Single-Fraction Radiotherapy to the Upper Abdomen. Priestman [32] demonstrated in his nonrandomized study with ondansetron that 4 mg 6-hourly or 8 mg 8-hourly achieved complete or major control of vomiting in 77–91% of patients, and mild or no nausea in 72–77% following single treatments to the upper abdomen. This was followed by a double-blind prospective randomized trial comparing 8 mg ondansetron 3 × day with 10 mg metoclopramide day for the prevention of emesis after single radiation doses of 8–10 Gy to the upper abdomen. There was complete control of emesis in 50% of patients with metoclopramide and in 75% with ondansetron. On days 2–5, there was no longer any statistically significant difference between ondansetron and metoclopramide, which may be related to a reduced emetic effect of radiotherapy at later time points, in contrast to chemotherapy. Nausea was less well controlled than emesis.

Hemibody Irradiation. Roberts and Priestman [37] performed a pilot study, using a combination of 8 mg ondansetron and 8 mg dexamethasone prior to treatment. They evaluated 11 patients with upper HBI using a single 6-Gy fraction and one patient with lower HBI using 8 Gy. They achieved 86% complete control of emesis with this combination. In 1992, Scarantino et al. [39] also showed excellent control of emesis in upper and mid-HBI with ondansetron.

Total-Body Irradiation. There are several published studies concerning TBI-induced emesis, as it is the most emetogenic radiotherapeutic regimen. Despite the use of optimal non-5-HT$_3$ receptor antagonist antiemetics, such as metoclopramide, emesis and nausea are almost universal after TBI and are equally prevalent whether treatment is given as a single dose or as a fractionated course with doses as low as 1.2 Gy daily [47].

Prentice et al. [31] randomized 30 patients into two groups receiving either granisetron or a combination of metoclopramide, dexamethasone, and lorazepam. After 24 h, emesis was completely controlled in 53% of those receiving granisetron, but in only 13% of those treated with the comparator regimen. Belkacémi et al. [3] investigated 36 patients receiving single-dose TBI before bone marrow transplantation. The patients received granisetron before TBI using two different modalities. Gibbs and Cassoni [18] examined the duration of antiemetic effect of granisetron in a pilot study of patients ($n = 26$) undergoing a standard emetogenic stimulus in the form of TBI fractionated over 3–4 days in a randomized comparison with twice-daily ondansetron. Croockewit [7] treated 21 patients with TBI after high-dose cyclophosphamide. Complete or major control of emesis was achieved in 71–95% during TBI and in 82–95% in the 5 days following TBI.

Kaasa et al. [27] used ondansetron during TBI with 1.3 Gy twice daily over a period of 5 days. They achieved 50–80% complete or good control of emesis and nausea during TBI with ondansetron, and 55–80% reported nausea as nonexistent or mild on each day. In 1994, Spitzer [45] performed a randomized double-blind, placebo-controlled evaluation of oral ondansetron in the prevention of nausea and vomiting: 20 patients who received 4 days of TBI were randomized to receive either 8-mg oral doses of ondansetron or placebo with ondansetron used as rescue. All patients initially treated with placebo required rescue with i.v. ondansetron, and six were subsequently controlled, while in 60% of those treated with prophylactic oral ondansetron emesis was controlled throughout their TBI. Results from these studies are summarized in Table 4.

Conventional Daily Fractionated Radiotherapy to the Abdominal Region. A recently completed study showed that approximately 40% of patients experienced emesis and nausea when undergoing fractionated radiotherapy between thorax and pelvis without antiemetic prophylaxis [12].

There are several studies comparing the efficacy of 5-HT$_3$ antagonists and conventional antiemetics. Priestman and his group compared the safety and efficacy of ondansetron and prochlorperazine in patients receiving multiple daily fractions of radiotherapy to the upper abdomen [34, 35, 37]. They found that 61% of patients prescribed ondansetron and 35% of those given prochlorperazine had a complete response with no emetic episodes in the whole of their treatment course. When control of emesis was evaluated according to the number of fractions of radiotherapy received, ondansetron provided complete control in a greater proportion of patients than prochlorperazine irrespective of the length of fractionated treatment. Furthermore, a significantly greater proportion of emesis-free days was observed in the ondansetron-treated patients than in those receiving prochlorperazine.

Table 4 Trials of 5-HT$_3$ receptor antagonists for emesis control in patients undergoing TBI (*RET* retrospective, *PRO* prospective, *CY* cyclophosphamide, *OND* ondansetron, *GRA* granisetron, *TBI* total-body irradiation, *CR* complete response, *MR* major response, *MEL* melphalan, *NS* not specified; from [43])

Reference	Center	Trial design	No. of patients	Conditioning regimen	Drug	Dose	Outcome
[24]	Hospital for Sick Children Bristol, UK	RET	15	CY 120 mg/kg ⇒TBI 1.8 Gy b.i.d. at 0.2 Gy/min × 4 days	OND	5 mg/m^2 i.v. q 8 h × 7 days	93% CR or MR
[25]	Royal Free Hospital, London	RET	32	TBI 7.5 Gy at 0.5 ± 0.02 Gy/min	GRA	40 µg/kg prior to TBI	97% CR or MR
[26]	Universität Kinderklinik, Münster, Germany	RET	15	NS	OND	2.4 or 8 mg i.v. t.d.s. on "worst" TBI day	57% CR (vomiting) 86% CR or MR (nausea)
[41]	Berlin	RET	25	TBI 2.0 Gy b.i.d. or 4.0 Gy q.d.s. × 3 days	OND	5 mg/m^2 before TBI (additional two doses as required)	
[47]	Royal Marsden, London	PRO	20	MEL 110 mg/m^2 TBI 10.5 Gy at 0.04 Gy/min	Phenobarbitone + corticosteroids ± OND	8 mg i.v. before TBI	Fewer emetic episodes ($p = 0.029$) compared with placebo
[44]	Georgetown, Washington, DC	PRO	20	TBI 13.2 Gy at 0.22 Gy/min in 11 fractions over 4 days	OND (versus placebo)	8 mg p.o. before each TBI dose	Fewer emetic episodes ($p = 0.005$) Delayed time of onset ($p = 0.003$) compared with placebo
[13]	Universität Leipzig	RET	59 (35 vs 24)	TBI (2.0 Gy b.i.d. × 3 days) CY 60 mg/m^2 (2 days)	OND vs MCP	8 mg i.v. before TBI + 8 mg dexamethasone	90–97% CR, MR 54% CR, MR

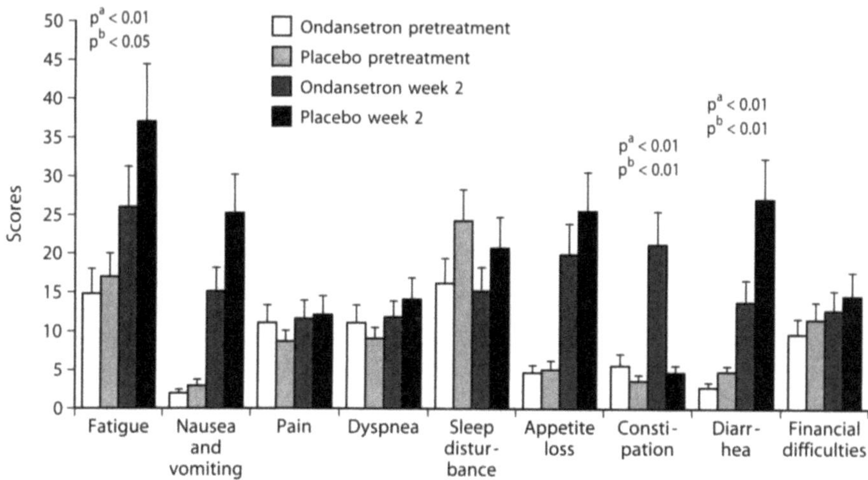

Fig. 5 EORTC QLQ C-30 symptom scales and items. Mean standard error at pretreatment check and at week 2 (higher score = more or more severe symptoms) [16]

Sorbe et al. [42] evaluated tropisetron as antiemetic prophylaxis during postoperative abdominal irradiation of ovarian cancer patients. The efficacy of tropisetron was rated excellent or good in 80% of cases. The overall ratings for quality of life were excellent or good in 75–85% of cases.

In 1996, Franzen et al. [16] reported the results of a randomized placebo-controlled study with ondansetron in patients undergoing fractionated radiotherapy to the abdomen: 111 patients about to commence a course of at least ten daily treatments were included. Of those receiving ondansetron, 67% had complete control of emesis, as against 45% of patients with placebo. This study also assessed quality of life and showed benefits for patients receiving ondansetron during radiotherapy (Fig. 5).

The value of tropisetron for control of nausea and vomiting and as rescue therapy was studied by Mirabell et al. [30]. A total of 88 patients who were undergoing fractionated radiotherapy to the abdomen or to large supradiaphragmatic fields and had failed a first antiemetic trial with metoclopramide were included.

Henriksson et al. [23] reported on 33 patients receiving fractionated upper abdominal irradiation to fields larger than 100 cm^2 and receiving 1.8–4 Gy daily. They were treated with 8 mg oral ondansetron every 8 h. Emesis was completely controlled in 79% of patients.

Feyer [14] reported a series of 94 patients at moderate emetogenic risk (radiotherapy to the upper abdominal region) who were treated with prophylactic ondansetron. There was complete control in 84%, between two and five emetic episodes in 16% and failure in 6% of patients. A comparable patient group treated with conventional antiemetics, mostly metoclopramide, showed only 43% complete control, demonstrating almost 50% improvement with ondansetron.

Conclusions

The introduction of 5-HT$_3$ receptor antagonists resulted in a dramatic improvement in the control of emesis, whether caused by chemotherapy or radiotherapy. There are only few published studies with radiotherapy, but the benefits are clear, especially in highly emetogenic regimens such as TBI. The use of 5-HT$_3$ receptor antagonists will also improve the quality of life in patients receiving emetogenic radiation therapy [46].

The choice of 5-HT$_3$ receptor antagonist and the optimal dosage in radiation-induced emesis are still subjects of debate, and the value of combination therapy, especially with dexamethasone, needs further evaluation.

Which patients undergoing radiotherapy require 5-HT$_3$ receptor antagonists? When selecting appropriate antiemetic therapy, the potential risk of emesis must first be assessed. For low-risk patients, it may be appropriate to start with a non-5-HT$_3$ antagonist, such as metoclopramide, alizapride, or chlorpromazine (Table 5). An alternative approach, for low- or medium-risk patients, is to use interventional antiemetics in patients who vomit. This approach does work, and studies have recently been completed that show the value of tropisetron and ondansetron in this manner [30]. This approach will provide adequate control at reasonable cost.

The basic principles of antiemetic therapy in radiotherapy should be:
- Prophylaxis as a therapeutic principle
- Antiemetic regimen selected with due consideration for the emetogenic risk
- Combined therapy in high-risk patients
- When appropriate, regular administration of antiemetics rather than administration on demand

Optimal selection of antiemetic prophylaxis and therapy should be an established part of supportive therapy and must be integrated into the planning of radiotherapy in order to improve the therapeutic outcome and especially the patients' quality of life.

Table 5 Indications for the use of antiemetics depending on the emetogenic risk during radiotherapy

Emetogenic potential of radiotherapy	Risk profile of the patient	Antiemetic prophylaxis
Mild	Normal	None
	High	None
Moderate	Normal	None
	High	Non-5-HT$_3$ antagonists or 5-HT$_3$ antagonists (p.o.)
Severe	Normal	5-HT$_3$ antagonists (p.o./i.v.) or
	High	5-HT$_3$ antagonists + dexamethasone (i.v.) ± sedation

Consensus Statement

1. Depending on the emetogenic potential of the radiotherapy and the individual risk profile of the patient, the prophylaxis of emesis should be an integral part of the treatment planning.
   Level of consensus:　　　Moderate
   Level of confidence:　　　Not applicable

2. Radiotherapy to the lower thorax, abdomen, or pelvis is potentially emetogenic (especially when large volumes are irradiated). Hemibody irradiation that includes the upper abdomen is highly emetogenic.
   Level of consensus:　　　High
   Level of confidence:　　　High

3. The dose administered and pattern of fractionation are also important factors in determining the degree of emesis.
   Level of consensus:　　　Moderate
   Level of confidence:　　　Not applicable

4. Studies using non-5-HT$_3$ receptor antagonist antiemetics demonstrate moderate control (approx. 50%) for moderately emetogenic radiotherapy but only poor control for highly emetogenic radiotherapy.
   Level of consensus:　　　High
   Level of confidence:　　　High

5. Comparative studies show improved control when 5-HT$_3$ receptor antagonist antiemetics are used with moderate and highly emetogenic radiotherapy.
   Level of consensus:　　　High
   Level of confidence:　　　High

6. For moderately emetogenic daily fractionated radiotherapy, interventional therapy is effective but must be commenced as soon as symptoms (usually nausea) develop. Non-5-HT$_3$ receptor antagonists may be effective, but there is good evidence for the efficacy of 5-HT$_3$ receptor antagonists in this situation.
    Level of consensus: Moderate
    Level of confidence: High

7. There is a small group of patients who receive highly emetogenic radiotherapy. These patients should receive 5-HT$_3$ receptor antagonist antiemetics as prophylaxis prior to commencing radiotherapy.
    Level of consensus: High
    Level of confidence: High

8. The addition of dexamethasone may improve control of emesis for moderately and highly emetogenic radiotherapy.
    Level of consensus: Moderate
    Level of confidence: Moderate

9. There is clear consensus for the use of 5-HT$_3$ receptor antagonist antiemetics (with or without dexamethasone) for highly and moderately emetogenic radiotherapy, but further studies are required to determine optimal antiemetic regimens for moderately emetogenic daily fractionated radiotherapy.
    Level of consensus: High
    Level of confidence: Not applicable

10. Total-body irradiation together with high-dose chemotherapy is usually given over several days and is a highly emetogenic combination. The combination of a 5-HT$_3$ receptor antagonist antiemetic and dexamethasone will provide optimal emesis control for both the irradiation and the chemotherapy.
    Level of consensus: High
    Level of confidence: Moderate

11. Further studies are required to determine optimal dosing and timing and to find out whether combination therapy, including benzodiazepines, is more effective than 5-HT$_3$ receptor antagonists alone. In this particular setting, it is difficult to determine the incidence and severity of delayed emesis related to radiotherapy and chemotherapy owing to other compounding factors that may produce emesis, e.g., reinfusion of stem cells, antibiotic and antifungal therapy.
    Level of consensus: High
    Level of confidence: Not applicable

References

1. Anno GH, Baum SJ, Withers HR, Young RW (1989) Symptomatology of acute radiation effects in humans after exposure to doses of 0.5–30 Gy. Health Phys 56 : 821–838
2. Barret A (1982) Total body irradiation (TBI) before bone marrow transplantation in leukaemia: a cooperative study from the European Group for Bone Marrow Transplantation. Br J Radiol 55 : 562–570
3. Belkacémi Y, Ozsahin M, Pène F, Rio B, Sutton L, Laporte JP, Touboul E, Gorin NC, Laugier A (1996) Total body irradiation prior to bone marrow transplantation: efficacy and safety of granisetron in the prophylaxis and control of radiation-induced emesis. Int J Radiat Oncol Biol Phys 36 : 77–82
4. Blower PR (1990) The role of specific 5-HT$_3$-receptor antagonsim in the control of cytostatic drug-induced emesis. Eur J Cancer 26 [Suppl 1] : 8–11
5. Bremer K (1994) Individuelle risikoadaptierte antiemetische Stufentherapie. Dtsch Med Wochenschr 119 : 598–604
6. Buell MG, Harding RK (1989) Proinflammatory effects of local irradiation on the rat gastrointestinal tract. Dig Dis Sci 34 : 390–399
7. Croockewit S (1990) The efficacy of ondansetron in emesis induced by total body irradiation (abstract). ESMO, Satellite Symposium on Zofran, pp 15–17
8. Court-Brown WM (1953) Symptomatic disturbance after single therapeutic dose of x-rays. Br J Med I : 802–805
9. Coates A, Abraham SK, Kaye SB (1983) On the receiving end: patient perception of the side effects of cancer chemotherapy. Eur J Cancer Clin Oncol 19 : 203
10. Danjoux E, Rider WD, Fritzpatrick PJ (1979) The acute radiation syndrome. Clin Radiol 30 : 581–584
11. Davis CJ, Harding RK, Leslie RA, Andrews PLR (1986) The organization of vomiting as a protective reflex. In: Davis CJ, Lake-Bakaar GV, Grahame-Smith DG (eds) Nausea and vomiting: mechanisms and treatment. Springer, Berlin Heidelberg New York, pp 65–75
12. Feyer PC (1994) Incidence of emesis and nausea in fractionated radiotherapy patients. In: Advances in optimising the control of emesis. Satellite Symposium to ESMO, Lisbon, November 1994
13. Feyer P (1994) Investigations comparing acute reactions and late effects of different conditioning regimens prior to bone marrow transplantation. Thesis. University of Leipzig
14. Feyer P (1995) Ondansetron in radiotherapy-induced emesis. J Pharmacol Ther 4 : 112–113
15. Fowler J, Lindstrom M (1992) Loss of local control with prolongation in radiotherapy. Int J Radiat Oncol Biol Phys 23 : 457–467
16. Franzen L, Nyman I, Hagberg H, Jakobsson M, Sorbe B, Nyth AL, Lomberg H, Henriksson R (1996) A randomised placebo controlled study with ondansetron in patients undergoing fractionated radiotherapy. Am Oncol 7 : 587–592
17. Gagnon GJ, Kuettel M (1994) Diurnal variation in acute GI-toxicity from prostate cancer radiotherapy. Proc Am Soc Ther Radiol Oncol 1018 : 253
18. Gibbs SJ, Cassoni AM (1996) A pilot study to evaluate the cost effectiveness of ondansetron and granisetron in fractionated total body irradiation. Clin Oncol 8 : 182–184
19. Harding RK (1995) 5-HT$_3$ receptor antagonists and radiation-induced emesis: preclinical data. In: Reynolds DJM, Andrews PLR, Davis CJ (eds) Serotonin and the

scientific basis of antiemetic therapy, chap 12. (Oxford clinical communications) Oxford University Press, Oxford, pp 127–133

20. Harding RK, Leach KE, Prud`homme-Lalonde L, Ferrarotto CL (1991) Release of inflammatory mediators from irradiated gastrointestinal tissues. Gastroenterology 98 : A285

21. Harding RK, Morris GP, Prud´homme-Lalonde L, Leach KE (1992) Acute effects of 5 Gy ionizing irradiation on mast cell populations in the ferret jejunum. Gastroenterology 102 : A635

22. Harding RK, Young RW, Anno GH (1993) Radiotherapy-induced emesis. In: Andrews PLR, Sanger GJ (eds) Emesis in anticancer therapy mechanisms and treatment, chap 8. Chapman and Hall, London, pp 163–178

23. Henriksson R, Lomberg H, Isrealsson G, Zackrisson B, Franzen L (1992) The effect of ondansetron on radiation-induced emesis and diarrhoea. Acta Oncol 31 : 767–769

24. Hewitt M, Cornish J, Pamphilon D, Oakhill A (1991) Effective emetic control during conditioning of children for bone marrow transplantation using ondansetron, a 5-HT$_3$ antagonist. Bone Marrow Transplant 7 : 431–433

25. Hunter AE, Prentice HG, Pothecary K (1991) Granisetron, a selective 5HT$_3$-receptor antagonist for the prevention of radiation-induced emesis during total body irradiation. Bone Marrow Transplant 7 : 439–441

26. Jürgens H, McQuade B (1992) Ondansetron as prophylaxis for chemotherapy and radiotherapy induced emesis in children. Oncology 49 : 279–285

27. Kaasa S, Kvaly S, Lauvvang G (1993) The role of ondansetron in patients receiving total body irradiation (abstract). Seventh ECCO: Progress in the Management of Emesis, Jerusalem, Israel, 14-18 November 1993

28. Krook JE, Moertel CG, Gunderson LL (1991) Effective surgical adjuvant therapy for high risk rectal carcinoma. N Engl J Med 324 : 709

29. Lucraft HH, Palmer MK (1982) Randomized clinical trial of levanantradol and chlorpromazine in prevention of radiotherapy-induced vomiting. Clin Radiol 33 : 621–622

30. Mirabell R, Coucke P, Behrouz F, Blazek N, Melliger M, Philipps S, Wickenhauser R, Gebhard S, Schwabb T, Rosset A (1995) Nausea and vomiting in fractionated radiotherapy: a prospective on-demand trial of tropisetron rescue for non-responders to metoclopramide. Eur J Cancer [A] 31 : 1461–1464

31. Prentice GH, Cunningham S, Gandhi L, Cunningham J, Collis C, Hamon MD (1995) Granisetron in the prevention of irradiation-induced emesis. Bone Marrow Transplant 15 : 445–448

32. Priestman TJ (1989) Clinical studies with ondansetron in the control of radiation-induced emesis. Eur J Cancer Clin Oncol 251 : 29–33

33. Priestman TJ, Priestman SG (1984) An initial evaluation of nabilone in the control of radiotherapy induced nausea and vomiting. Clin Radiol 35 : 265–266

34. Priestman TJ, Roberts JT, Upadhyaya BK (1992) Randomised double-blind trial of ondansetron and prochlorperazine in the prevention of fractionated radiotherapy induced emesis. Proc Am Soc Clin Oncol 9 : 1370

35. Priestman TJ, Roberts JT, Upadhyaya BK (1993) A prospective randomized double-blind trial comparing ondansetron versus prochlorperazine for the prevention of nausea and vomiting in patients undergoing fractionated radiotherapy. Clin Oncol 5 : 358–363

36. Reyntjens R (1979) Domperidone as an anti-emetic: summary of research reports. Postgrad Med J 55 : 50–54

37. Roberts JT, Priestmann TJ (1993) A review of ondansetron in the management of radiotherapy induced emesis. Oncology 50 : 173–179

38. Robertson A, Robertson C, Symonds R (1993) Effect of varying schedules on carcinoma of the larynx. Eur J Cancer 29 : 501–510
39. Scarantino CW, Ornitz RD, Hoffmann LG, Anderson RF (1992) Radiation-induced emesis: effects of ondansetron. Semin Oncol 6 [Suppl 15] : 38–43
40. Scarantino CW, Ornitz RD, Hoffman LG, Anderson RF (1993) On the mechanism of radiation-induced emesis. The role of serotonin. Int J Radiat Oncol Biol Phys 27 [Suppl 1] : 159
41. Schwella N, König V, Schwerdtfeger R, Schmidt-Wolf I, Schmid H, Riess H, Siegert W (1994) Ondansetron for efficient emesis control during total body irradiation. Bone Marrow Transplant 13 : 169–171
42. Sorbe B, Berglind AM, Bruijn K de (1992) Tropisetron, a new 5-HT$_3$-receptor antagonist, in the prevention of radiation-induced emesis. Radiother Oncol 2 : 131–132
43. Spitzer TR (1995) Clinical evidence for 5-HT3 receptor antagonist efficacy in radiation-induced emesis. In: Reynolds DJM, Andrews PLR, Davis CJ (eds) Serotonin and the scientific basis of antiemetic therapy. (Oxford clinical communications) Oxford University Press, Oxford, pp 134-141
44. Spitzer TR, Deeg HJ, Torrisi J (1990) Total body irradiation-induced emesis is universal after small dose fractions (120 cGy) and is not cumulative dose related. Proc Am Soc Clin Oncol 9 : 14
45. Spitzer TR, Bryson JC, Cirenza E (1994) Randomized double-blind, placebo-controlled evaluation of oral ondansetron in the prevention of nausea and vomiting associated with fractionated total body irradiation. J Clin Oncol 12 : 2432–2435
46. Sykes A, Kiltie A Stewart A (1997) Ondansetron versus a chlorpromazine and dexamethasone combination for the prevention of nausea and vomiting; a prospective, randomised study to assess the efficacy, costeffectiveness and quality of life in patients following single fraction radiotherapy. Support Care Cancer 5 : 500-503
47. Tiley C, Powles R, Caatalano J, Treleaven J, Eshelby J, Hewetson M, Tait D, Cunningham D (1992) Results of a double blind placebo controlled study of ondansetron as an antiemetic during total body irradiation in patients undergoing bone marrow transplantation. Leuk Lymphoma 7 : 317–321
48. Westbrook C, Glasholm J, Barrett A (1987) Vomiting associated with whole body irradiation. Clin Radiol 38 : 263–266

Statistical Considerations in the Design, Conduct, and Analysis of Antiemetic Clinical Trials

An Emerging Consensus

Gary R. Morrow, Enzo Ballatori, Susan Groshen, Ian Olver

ABSTRACT Various aspects of trial design and planning for clinical testing of antiemetic therapies administered to cancer patients are considered. It is generally felt that a randomized double-blind parallel-arm design is the best. Ways of achieving adequate power of such studies are discussed briefly, as is the need for previous identification of primary and secondary end points. Finally, summary recommendations are given.

Introduction

A number of recent summaries have described desirable features of the planning, design, and analysis of antiemetic trials in patients being treated for cancer [1, 3, 5, 10, 17, 19, 20]. In phase III testing, a consensus has emerged that the optimum design is a randomized double-blind parallel-arm design. The study must have adequate power to detect clinically meaningful differences. Stratification by previously identified prognostic factors could be considered. Adequately measured primary and secondary end points need to be clearly identified in advance. These specific points are described more fully below.

Randomization

Randomization distributes known and unknown prognostic factors among the arms of a trial in an unbiased manner, so that the effects of these prognostic factors are averaged out in tests of statistical significance [21]. Randomization avoids the conscious or subconscious assignment of certain patients to particular arms of a study. Nonrandomized designs are unacceptable for phase III comparative antiemetic trials.

Double Blind

Every effort should be made to double blind all comparative antiemetic trials, since both nausea and vomiting may be influenced by external stimuli and suggestion as well as the direct emetogenic effect of the chemotherapy, and because nausea is self-reported. However, it must be recognized that blinding may be difficult to achieve. Informed consent information that describes different side effects for different arms of the study may make blinding difficult. If the drugs being compared have differing side effects, both patients and treating staff may be able to accurately ascertain one or more of the arms [23]. If subjective criteria are used, it is essential that maximum efforts be made to ensure that at least the patient is blinded to the treatment assignment.

Parallel Design

A parallel design should be chosen for antiemetic studies. A crossover design is intuitively appealing and has been successfully used in a variety of fields. The crossover design is often advocated because it allows for patient preference, avoids interpatient variability, and requires a smaller sample size. In the context of antiemetic studies, however, the latter two assumptions are likely to be false [12]. Because the second course of treatment may be different from the first course, the intrapatient variability may be no less than the interpatient variability. And since, in a crossover antiemetic trial, it is advisable to test for period and carry-over effects, the planned sample size may be greater than with a parallel study.

A further challenge to study integrity in a crossover design is the high probability of a substantial patient loss between subsequent chemotherapy cycles. With a crossover design, it is also not possible to evaluate the antiemetic efficacy over multiple cycles. Finally, there are also ethical and clinical concerns about changing a treatment that has been successful in the first period.

Stratification for Prognostic Factors

There is an emerging consensus that prognostic variables influence the outcome of antiemetic studies. Age, gender, prior long-term exposure to alcohol, and prior chemotherapy experience are generally considered to be strongly associated with nausea and vomiting. There is less consistent evidence for patient susceptibility to motion, patient anxiety, and setting of the

Table 1 Total number of patients needed for comparison of two antiemetic regimens (2-sided, $p<0.05$ Chi-squared test with 80% power)

% Complete control with "standard"	5% Improvement	10% Improvement	15% Improvement
40%	3146	814	372
60%	3020	752	330
80%	1890	438	176

chemotherapy [18]. There are probably further unexplored prognostic factors, such as emotional state, and as yet unexplored interactions among prognostic factors. Known and suspected factors should be prospectively assessed and evaluated as part of large antiemetic trials. Subgroup analysis based on these characteristics should be planned in order to further understand their potential role.

The aim of stratification prior to randomization is to assure a balance of known prognostic factors among experimental groups. When the sample size is sufficiently large, imbalance among experimental groups is unlikely. If interim analyses are planned, stratification prior to randomization should be more seriously considered because of the possibility that the trial may end early, which could result in a larger imbalance of characteristics among arms. However, if the sample size is sufficiently large and analyses are planned in advance, both stratification at the time of randomization and stratification at the time of analyses may be equally effective.

Sample Size

Sample sizes should be calculated to achieve adequate power (at least 80%; 90% is preferable) to detect differences that would be clinically meaningful. Although a large improvement may be expected (or hoped for), the study should be designed with the more modest, but still clinically relevant difference in mind. With the improved control of acute emesis with 5-HT$_3$ receptor antagonists, an improvement of 15% or smaller may be clinically important. This will serve to increase the required sample size.

Table 1 illustrates the interrelationships among the percent complete control with a standard or comparison antiemetic agent, the percent improvement desired to be detected, and the sample size needed to detect the improvement with a two-sided Chi-squared, test at a $p<0.05$ level and 80% power. The number of patients increases as the size of improvement to be detected decreases.

Studies designed to show equivalence of regimens should have greater power: 90% or more is recommended [6, 16]. In reporting of results, the criteria used for sample size determination should be reported, i.e., the desired power and what was considered a clinically important difference.

Interim Analyses

The timing of interim analyses should be preplanned so that the trial is not stopped early with a spuriously positive result. The probability of achieving $p=0.05$ by chance alone where no significant result actually exists can exceed 20% if interim analyses are performed every 6 months in a 4-year study [2]. Termination of a trial prior to the target sample size requires a p value smaller than 0.05 [9, 11, 24].

Intent-to-Treat Analysis

If not all randomized patients are adequately treated and evaluable, an intent-to-treat analysis must be performed [12, 23]. An intent-to-treat analysis requires that all patients who were assigned to a regimen be included in the denominator of the estimates of efficacy of that regimen. If an "as-treated" analysis is also performed, the results of that analysis should be compared with the results of the intent-to-treat analysis [15]. All patients who are randomized should be accounted for [14].

Selection of End Points

End points must be clearly defined before the trial begins. Nausea and vomiting should be separately evaluated, not only because of the dependence of nausea and vomiting on different physiopathological mechanisms, but also to distinguish any different efficacy of antiemetic therapies for nausea and vomiting [7, 18, 22]. While the occurrence and severity of nausea and vomiting are of primary clinical interest, symptom duration may provide important additional information.

An analysis of the association between nausea and vomiting is recommended to evaluate whether the presence of nausea can explain or account for the relationship between the different efficacy of the antiemetic treatments and the protection from vomiting.

Issues for the Design of Future Trials

Methodological challenges remain in exploring unresolved issues, including: treatment of patients for whom initial antiemetic therapy has failed; control of delayed emesis; prevention of emesis on repeated courses of chemotherapy; tailoring therapies to subsets of patients (giving less therapy for those at lower risk of emesis and more therapy for those at greater risk); identifying effective regimens that can be delivered on an outpatient basis; combining drugs and altering schedules to further improve the control of emesis. Future trials will involve assessment beyond the initial 24 h and include several courses. Sample size calculations will need to consider the number of patients treated and observed at later courses as well as at the first course.

Studies of Delayed Emesis

Delayed nausea or vomiting should be described considering both (1) the day-by-day response, e.g., the severity from each day measured separately, in order to evaluate the pattern of the phenomenon, and (2) a summary measurement for the whole period, e.g., the maximum emesis observed on day 1 or during days 2–6, or the time until emesis is first observed. Both approaches will be useful in comparisons and evaluation of potential relationship(s) between delayed emesis and potentially prognostic factors.

A dependence of delayed emesis on acute emesis may contribute to differences in observed efficacy between acute and delayed side effects. The association between emesis during the first 24 h and the delayed emesis should be summarized by the type of antiemetic and the type of chemotherapy treatment given the patient [13]. Comparative trials should be specifically designed to evaluate delayed emesis. The treatment of acute emesis should be administered in a standard manner. One approach is to randomize patients prior to any treatment and perform an intent-to-treat analysis. This allows evaluation both of patients who experience little or no acute emesis prior to the experience of delayed emesis and of those patients who experience severe emesis during the acute phase.

In studies where patients are randomized after the acute phase, stratification should be based on a patient's response during the acute phase. It is important to record information on those patients who drop out because of acute nausea/emesis. In the situation that all the patients receive the same prophylaxis against delayed emesis, some information regarding the different efficacy of the various regimens against delayed emesis can also be obtained.

Studies of Multiple Cycles of Chemotherapy

The analysis of multiple cycles of chemotherapy is complicated because of the dependence of each cycle on previous cycles. Furthermore, there may be a potential overlapping of acute and delayed emesis (and, depending on time between cycles, a potential overlap between delayed side effects of one cycle and anticipatory side effects of the next [17]). Statistical models need to describe nausea/vomiting over multiple cycles, allowing for the effect of dropouts on the observed treatment efficacy as well as a potential effect on prognostic factors [4]. In summarizing the results of a trial of multiple cycles, the following should be reported: the number of dropouts at each cycle, the reasons for their exclusion, and a summary of the primary prognostic factors.

Alternate Designs

Future studies will involve the comparison of combinations of two or more drugs, different schedules or routes of administration, or different doses. For these, factorial designs [8] will allow us to ask two or more questions simultaneously and have two important features: fewer patients are required than in the sequence of separate trials, each asking a single question; and interactions (synergy or antagonism) between treatment factors can be identified. If the goal is to select the best regimen (i.e., the best combination of treatment factors), then methods for statistical selection can be employed [4] in the setting of the factorial design. With selection methods, the regimen that achieves the best observed response is selected for use or for further study, or the two (or three) regimens with the best observed responses are selected for further study. The number of patients required is determined by probability requirement for correct selection. Methods of statistical selection have the advantage of generally requiring fewer patients than formal hypothesis-testing procedures. However, the individual questions (of scheduling, of dosing, etc.) are not addressed specifically and the regimen selected is not "proven" to be best, as is the case in formal hypothesis testing. Two-stage and multiple-stage selection methods are also available, in which a number of regimens are eliminated at each stage, allowing more patients to be assigned to those regimens which appear more effective in the earlier stages. These can also be used in early-phase testing of drugs, to identify the most biologically active doses for further testing.

Recommendations

Articles such as those briefly reviewed and discussions at the consensus conference lead us to suggest the following recommendations for the conduct of clinical trials evaluating antiemetic therapy:

1. A randomized, parallel-arm, double-blind study is the preferred design to compare the efficacy of two or more antiemetic therapies.
2. There are factors that may influence the likelihood of emesis following chemotherapy that must be part of the study design:
   a) The prognostic factors of age, gender, long-term exposure to alcohol, and prior chemotherapy experience have consistently been found to influence nausea and vomiting.
   b) Other potential prognostic factors should be investigated prospectively as part of large antiemetic trials.
3. Complete response for vomiting and nausea should be the primary end points of antiemetic trials, and these should be evaluated separately. The association between nausea and vomiting and its relationship with treatment should be analyzed.
4. Sample sizes should be calculated to achieve adequate power (at least 80%; 90% is preferable) to detect clinically meaningful differences.
5. Interim analyses should be preplanned so that a trial is not stopped early with a spuriously positive result.
6. An intent-to-treat analysis should be performed, and all randomized patients should be accounted for.
7. For studies of delayed emesis, the criterion used to define delayed emesis should be stated and the relationship of delayed nausea/vomiting and acute nausea/emesis should be allowed for in the analysis.
8. Clinical trials should be designed to measure both nausea and vomiting over multiple cycles of chemotherapy, and the analysis should take into consideration that cycles are not independent. When reporting results, the number of patients who drop out at each cycle for each arm should be specified and the reasons for dropout should be summarized.

References

1. Aapro M (1993) Methodological issues in antiemetic studies. Invest New Drugs 11:243–253
2. Armitage PW, McPherson K, Rowe BC (1969) Repeated significance tests on accumulating data. Journal of the Royal Statistical Society A 132:235–244
3. Ballatori E, Roila F, Del Favero A (1996) Methodology of antiemetic trials. In: Tonato M (ed) Antiemetics in the supportive care in cancer. Springer, Berlin Heidelberg New York, pp 35–47

4. Bechhofer RE, Santner TJ, Goldsman DM (1995) Design and analysis of experiments for statistical selection, screening, and multiple comparisons. Wiley, New York

5. Bergmann JF (1995) Méthodologie de l'évaluation des antiémétiques. Bull Cancer 82:1062–1066

6. Blackwelder WC (1982) Proving the null hypothesis in clinical trials. Control Clin Trials 3:345–353

7. Bonneterre J, Hecquet B, Adenis A, Fournier C, Pion JM, Demaille A (1991) How do patients and physicians decide which antiemetic is the best in a cross-over study? Proc ASCO 10:323

8. Byar DP, Piantadosi S (1985) Factorial designs for randomized clinical trials. Cancer Treat Rep 69:1055–1063

9. Geller NL (1987) Planned interim analysis and its role in cancer clinical trials. J Clin Oncol 5:1857–1490

10. Gralla RJ, Clark RA, Kris MG, Tyson LB (1991) Methodology in anti-emetic trials. Eur J Cancer 27 [Suppl 1]:S5–S8

11. Green SJ, Fleming TR, O'Fallon JR (1987) Policies for study monitoring and interim reporting of results. J Clin Oncol 5:477–1484

12. Groshen S (1992) Antiemetic study design: a discussion of Dr. Olver's paper. Br J Cancer 66 [Suppl XIX]:S35–S37

13. Italian Group for Antiemetic Research (1997) Delayed emesis induced by moderate emetogenic chemotherapy: do we need to treat all patients? Ann Oncol (in press)

14. Lee YJ, Ellenberg JH, Hirtz DG, Nelson KB (1991) Analysis of clinical trials by treatment actually received: is it really an option? Stat Med 10:1595–1605

15. Lewis JA, Machin D (1993) Intention to treat – who should use ITT? Br J Cancer 68:647–650

16. Makuch R, Simon R (1978) Sample size requirements for evaluating a conservative therapy. Cancer Treat Rep 62:1037–1040

17. Morrow GR (1992) Methodology and assessment in clinical anti-emetic research: a meta-analysis of outcome parameters. Br J Cancer 66 [Suppl XIX]:S38–S41

18. Morrow GR, Roscoe JA (1997) Anticipatory nausea and vomiting: models, mechanisms and management. In: Dicato M (ed) Medical Management of Cancer-Treatment Induced Emesis. Martin Dunitz, London, pp 149-166

19. Olver IN (1992) Antiemetic study design: desirable objectives, stratifications and analyses. Br J Cancer 66 [Suppl XIX]:S30–S34

20. Olver IN (1996) Antiemetic study methodology: recommendations for future studies. Oncology 53 [Suppl 1]:96–101

21. Olver IN, Simon RM, Aisner J (1986) Antiemetic studies: a methodological discussion. Cancer Treat Rep 70:555–563

22. Olver IN, Matthews JP, Bishop JF, Smith RA (1994) The roles of patient and observer assessments in anti-emetic trials. Eur J Cancer [A] 30:1223–1227

23. Seipp CA, Chang AE, Shiling DJ, Rosenberg SA (1980) In search of an effective antiemetic: a nursing staff participates in marijuana research. Cancer Nurs 21:271–276

24. Zelen M (1987) Early stopping, interim analyses, and monitoring committees: what are the tradeoffs? J Clin Oncol 5:1314–1315

Neuropharmacology of Emesis and Its Relevance to Antiemetic Therapy
Consensus and Controversies

P. L. R. Andrews, R. J. Naylor, R. A. Joss

ABSTRACT Recent great advances in the neuropharmacology of the emetic pathways have led to better therapy and improved insight into pathophysiological processes in patients undergoing chemo- and radiotherapy. This article gives an overview of the area, outlines current controversies, and makes recommendations for future clinical studies.

Introduction

In the past decade, enormous advances have been made in our understanding of the neuropharmacology of the emetic pathways. These have led to improved antiemetic therapy and given important insights into the pathophysiological processes occurring in patients treated with cytotoxic drugs and radiation. This document is divided into three parts: (1) a general overview of the area based around aspects of the topic on which there is a large measure of consensus; (2) areas of controversy, uncertainty, and current research; (3) recommendations of clinical studies which would assist understanding of basic mechanisms.

Current Concepts of the Neuropharmacology of Emesis

The discovery [10, 22] that blockade of one subtype of the 5-hydroxytryptamine (5-HT) receptor, the 5-HT$_3$ receptor, could block the "acute" emetic response (retching and vomiting) induced by cisplatin in an animal model (ferret) was the key advance. In some ways this was a fortuitous event. Granisetron, ondansetron, and tropisetron, effectively abolished emesis observed over an acute 4-h period. If the authors had used a longer period of observation, then the relative resistance of the delayed phase would have revealed an incomplete control. This would surely have jeopardised the progression of such compounds to developmental status, ensuring their failure to reach the clinic, and would have relegated emesis research to obscurity. Such is life! The importance of the 5-HT$_3$ receptor antagonists is that they provided a precise pharmacological tool with which to study the pathways involved in cisplatin-induced emesis as a protypical cytotoxic drug. With the identification of the site of action of the 5-HT$_3$ receptor antagonists, the role of the vagal afferent-enterochromaffin cell (EC cell) functional unit in the emetic response was identified [5]. In addition, the introduction of 5-HT$_3$ receptor antagonists stimulated clinical research and improved the quantification of nausea and emesis.

The identification of the site of action of the 5-HT$_3$ receptor antagonists stimulated research into emetic mechanisms in general, and as a consequence there has been a major reappraisal of the relative involvement of the area postrema (AP, popularly referred to as the "chemoreceptor trigger zone for emesis") and the abdominal visceral afferents, particularly the vagus, and this continues (for reviews, see [1, 3]). In particular, the involvement of the AP in the emetic response to all systemic agents is a matter of debate. The recognition of the significance of the nucleus tractus solitarius (NTS, the main integrative nucleus for visceral and some somatic functions in the brain stem, subjacent to the AP) in emesis has grown in prominence, particularly the realization that the dendrites from the NTS neurons invade the AP [27]. Thus surgical ablation of the AP inevitably causes damage to these dendrites, some of which receive inputs from the abdominal vagal afferents terminating in the subnucleus gelatinosus of the NTS. Therefore, lesions directed at the area postrema may damage these vagal pathways and, if emesis is affected, may give rise to the erroneous conclusion that the AP was the primary site at which the emetic agent was acting (see [3] for a review).

The focus of the above mechanistic studies was the acute phase of emesis induced by cytotoxic drugs, as this is the most intense phase, but such studies need to be repeated in the recently described models of delayed emesis [16, 31, 33].

The application of electrophysiological and molecular techniques to emesis has provided novel insights into the action of cytotoxic drugs at the cellular level. For example, cisplatin acutely increases the excitability of cultured neurons at concentrations reported clinically, but chronic exposure produced complex effects indicative of interference with calcium homeostasis [35] (cf. proposed mechanisms of renal toxicity). Some of the chronic toxic effects of cisplatin were reduced by dexamethasone.

Studies by Matsuki et al. [19] have provided evidence showing that free radical generation is probably the key step in the mechanism by which cytotoxic drugs evoke the calcium-dependent exocytotic release of 5-HT from the ECs. This raises the question of why the ECs are so sensitive to cytotoxic drugs and radiation; if they were not, it is probable that emesis would be less of a problem with cytostatic agents.

Studies of the way in which the release of 5-HT is controlled have continued and appear to support the proposal that it involves a positive feedback via 5-HT$_3$ receptors. While there is some evidence for a negative feedback (saturating at low concentrations of 5-HT) via 5-HT$_4$ receptors, this is still a matter of debate (for reviews, see [25, 37]). Evidence from human studies supporting the hypothesis that cytotoxic drugs release 5-HT from the ECs has continued to accumulate, and further insights have been provided by the measurement of plasma chromogranin A [13]. However, an interesting anomaly has appeared with cyclophosphamide, where apart from the sensitivity of the emetic response to 5-HT$_3$ receptor antagonists, the urinary 5-HIAA, measurements provide no evidence for an involvement of 5-HT. This requires further investigation.

The activation of the early immediate oncogene *c-fos* has been used to map some of the central neuronal pathways involved in the emetic response to a range of emetic agents, including cisplatin [27]. These studies reveal that even when the emetic response is blocked by administration of a 5-HT$_3$ receptor antagonist, *c-fos* (an index of neuronal activation) activation still occurs in some brain stem regions, most notably the AP. This indicates that the AP may have a permissive role, or alternatively that an action here may be responsible for some of the other effects of the cytotoxic drugs, such as nausea, reduced food intake, and conditioned taste aversions, which are less affected by 5-HT$_3$ receptor antagonists than emesis. This observation should also serve to remind us that even if a patient does not have nausea or vomiting, the cytotoxic drug will still have damaging effects on the patient, which may be responsible for other deleterious effects.

The above brief outline of some of the key aspects of basic research gives an insight into the progress that has been made from a preclinical perspective. However, it would be erroneous to think that now that the 5-HT$_3$ receptor antagonists are well established clinically throughout the world, basic studies no longer have a place (see below).

Controversial and Novel Areas

Are the Emetic Pathways in Man the Same as in Animals?

A Darwinian Approach to Emesis in Anticancer Therapy

Whilst it is impossible to answer this question by direct experimentation, a large body of circumstantial evidence supports the view that the vagus-EC cell functional unit plays a key role in the emetic response to cytotoxic drugs and radiation. Viewing the emetic reflex from an evolutionary view as a protective reflex also supports this view. In addition, from an evolutionary perspective, it is nausea rather than vomiting that serves to generate the aversive response, and it is well known that once anticipatory nausea and vomiting have developed they are difficult to treat. This preclinical observation leads to the conclusion that optimal antiemetic treatment (e.g., oral/i.v. 5-HT$_3$ receptor antagonist with a steroid) should be given on the first course of anticancer therapy and not reserved for patients who have failed on conventional antiemetics.

The Continuing Problem of Nausea

It is clear that nausea is much less effectively dealt with than vomiting by the 5-HT$_3$ receptor antagonists, although the reason for this is not clear. Nausea (the warning) is often considered to be induced by "low"-intensity activation of a pathway that, when more intensely activated, leads to retching and vomiting. The observation that nausea is less affected than vomiting by 5-HT$_3$ receptor antagonists suggests that the genesis of nausea may involve activation of additional pathways to the vagal afferent–EC unit.The AP would be a likely site, and such a mechanism is supported by the lack of effect of the 5-HT$_3$ receptor antagonist granisetron on cisplatin-induced *c-fos* expression in the ferret [27]. Because of the severe limitations of studying a subjective sensation in animals, mechanistic studies of nausea must be undertaken in man.

The recent studies by Miller et al. [21] provide an excellent beginning. Measuring human cortical activity (using noninvasive magnetic source imaging) during vestibular and ipecacuanha-induced nausea, they recorded a cortical locus in the inferior frontal gyrus that demonstrated a greater number of dipoles during intense than during milder nausea. Such changes were not recorded during other forms of sensory stimulation. Future studies using other emetogenic challenges and antiemetic regimens may help to elucidate the details of the cortical and other brain systems and finally the mechanisms involved in nausea (and emesis). The techniques may also allow for an objective rather than subjective assessment of nausea.

In connection with this, it appears that the value of ipecacuanha to nausea and emesis research is frequently overlooked and better use could be made of this agent. Thus ipecacuanha-induced nausea and emesis may be a particularly useful model to investigate the antiemetic actions of 5-HT$_3$ receptor antagonists. In animal models, ondansetron and other 5-HT$_3$ receptor antagonists exert a selective action to inhibit emesis induced by cytotoxic drugs, radiation, and ipecacuanha. The great advantage of using ipecacuanha in humans is that it can be safely used in human volunteers to assess the potency and antiemetic efficacy of 5-HT$_3$ receptor antagonists [23] and other antiemetics, such as the NK$_1$ receptor antagonists, and generally makes it possible to avoid the difficulties inherent in using cancer patients.

It remains unlikely that its mode of action precisely reflects that of cytotoxic drugs.

Are There Animal Models of Patients?

When apparent differences are described between humans and animals, the phrase often used is "species differences". However, this does not explain what is involved and is often used to suggest that the data from the nonhuman animal is "wrong". This is a patently unsupportable view, and particularly so when such an phylogenetically ancient and significant protective reflex as emesis is being considered. In studying the response of animals to cytotoxic drugs or radiation, we are essentially studying the basic reflex pathways, primarily at the level of the brain stem. While this has provided key insights into pathways, as exemplified by the use of 5-HT$_3$ receptor antagonists, the limitations of such models must be borne in mind in assessment of the insights they provide into the mechanisms operating in cancer patients who are undergoing therapy.

One important aspect that needs to be addressed in comparing pathways in man and animals is the role of the cerebral cortex. There is little doubt that the cerebral cortex and related structures provide an important modulatory input to the brain stem, probably at both conscious and subconscious levels. In animals, it is impossible to assess the role of the cortex. However, it is not unreasonable to suppose that, except perhaps in the highest nonhuman primates, there is little conscious input in terms of "rationalizing" the experience. What is meant here is not that the animals do not find the experience distressing to some degree, but that they do not contextualize it, which must add to the globally stressful nature of the experience. In most of the animal studies, it is therefore the basic reflex mechanism of emesis induced by cytotoxic drugs and radiation that is being studied, rather than chemotherapy and radiotherapy. These mechanisms may be further modified by the presence of the tumor and concomitant medication, neither of which is present in the animal models.

Why Do Patients "Fail" on 5-HT$_3$ Receptor Antagonists in the Acute Phase of Emesis?

Provided that an adequate dose of a long-lasting 5-HT$_3$ receptor antagonist has been given, then "failure" cannot be attributed to inadequate blockade of the receptor. One possible conclusion is that another receptor or pathway is involved. Animal studies have revealed that the emetic system shows a degree of "plasticity" [6, 20]. It is possible that patients who fail on 5-HT$_3$ receptor antagonists have a greater expression of this pathway than patients in whom the drugs are "successful". It is apparent from these experiments that clinical studies should be directed towards careful investigation of the failures so that the pharmacology of the non-5-HT$_3$ pathways can be elucidated. This could be achieved by systematic characterisation of the effect of well-defined pharmacological agents on these patients.

There remain major differences between drug action to antagonize the emetic effects of single drug challenges in animals or human volunteers and the nausea and emesis occurring in the cancer patient undergoing therapy. Thus, in man, visual, auditory, or olfactory stimuli, e.g., the sight, sound, or smell of someone being sick or the psychological stimuli of anxiety, can contribute to the occurrence and intensity of nausea and vomiting. The cancer itself, if causing obstruction in the lower or upper intestinal system, raised intracranial pressure, hypercalcemia, renal failure, pain, gastric irritation, etc., can all contribute to nausea and vomiting. Also, associated drug treatments, e.g., opioids, nonsteroidal anti-inflammatory agents, drug abuse, or alcohol, may all exacerbate nausea and vomiting. The more advanced the cancer, the greater their contribution. In palliative care units, the incidence of nausea/vomiting may be as high as 90% [9]. The contribution these many factors make to antiemetic drug treatments remains less than certain. However, given that various stimuli may contribute to the emesis induced by chemotherapy, the success of the 5-HT$_3$ receptor antagonists in completely controlling emesis in some 60–80% of patients during the acute phase is remarkable. Failure in the remaining patients during the acute phase may reflect the input of additional stimuli resistant to 5-HT$_3$ receptor blockade; this may also account for the less than adequate control of nausea and vomiting during the delayed phase. It should be borne in mind that even the failures are having less nausea and vomiting than if they had not received any antiemetic treatment.

While the involvement of 5-HT and 5-HT$_3$ receptors (peripheral and central) in emesis induced by anti-cancer therapies is well accepted, Cubeddu et al. have recently published an apparently anomalous piece of evidence but nevertheless one that may give a clue to other mechanisms [12, 13]. In man, a raised urinary level of 5-HIAA following cisplatin treatment has been taken to reflect a release of 5-HT from the ECs and hence support a role for 5-HT in emesis [12, 13]. However, although cyclophosphamide-induced emesis is affected by 5-HT$_3$ receptor antagonists in man and animals, cyclophosphamide fails to increase urinary 5-HT levels; it is imperative that further studies, using a much broader range of cytotoxic drugs and radiation, be carried out to substantiate a raised urinary 5-HIAA level with an emetic potential.

What Mechanisms Are Involved in Delayed Emesis?

Delayed emesis remains a problem, although the new animal models may provide rapid advances as the pathways and the pharmacology of this phase are investigated. However, as there have been relatively few studies of the physiological changes occurring in patients during the delayed phase, it is not clear how closely the animal models mimic man. The efficacy of conventional doses of metoclopramide in the delayed phase suggests that gut motility may be perturbed during this phase. It is proposed that detailed studies of gastrointestinal function be undertaken in patients. This may provide some insights into the mechanism of delayed emesis, but also, and of equal impor-tance, be of use in assessing the damage caused to the gut by the anticancer treatments, which can influence the patients' return to a normal diet.

Studies (Andrews, Bingham and Davidson, unpublished observations) have been undertaken in rats showing a long-lasting (4 days) reduction in gastric emptying following a single injection of cisplatin, but it is not clear how the effect comes about or whether this could contribute to delayed emesis. Recently, a ferret and a piglet model of delayed emesis have been published [16, 31], but as yet the pathways have not been investigated. Information is urgently needed about the pathways involved in these animal models, in order to identify therapeutic approaches to the outstanding problem of delayed emesis. While the animal models of delayed emesis may superficially resemble the condition seen in man, it is important that food intake, gastrointestinal tract, autonomic nervous system function, and tissue damage are monitored in man in the delayed phase, so that these can be compared with the events happening in the animals. It is highly likely that delayed nausea and vomiting are multifactorial, perhaps with different mechanisms operating at different times, but this has not been investigated experimentally in man.

It should be remembered that the poor efficacy of 5-HT$_3$ receptor antagonists in man in the delayed phase does not exclude a role for 5-HT, acting on some other receptor, in this phase of the response, and the piglet studies of [16] support such a proposal.

The Quest for the Perfect Antiemetic

The "holy grail" or "El Dorado" of antiemetic research has been the identification of an antiemetic agent that blocks the response to all stimuli. The reason for this is that it obviates the need to understand the precise mechanism or pathway by which a particular emetic stimulus acts, and obviously such an agent would have widespread clinical utility. Two approaches to this problem are highlighted below.

Continuing Involvement of 5-HT Receptors

Recognizing the involvement of 5-HT in the central components on the emetic pathway, one approach to reducing 5-HT function has come from the use of 5-HT_{1A} receptor ligands (agonists), e.g., 8-OH-DPAT, buspirone (currently used in psychiatry), flesinoxan, and lesopitron, which, in animals, can reduce motion-, copper sulphate-, and cisplatin-induced emesis [18, 24, 30, 32]. Activation of somatodendritic 5-HT_{1A} autoinhibitory receptors in the raphe nuclei reduces 5-HT cell firing and 5-HT release throughout the central serotonergic system. This argues for an important role of central 5-HT mechanisms to modulate the emetic reflex. The clinical value of such agents, administered with or without 5-HT_3 receptor antagonists, is currently being assessed. Although initial clinical studies with buspirone have been disappointing [12], this may not be the optimal compound to use in testing the hypothesis.

Substance P and Its Receptor(s): A Way Forward?

In 1993, Andrews and Bhandari showed that the ultrapotent capsaicin analogue resinferatoxin (RTX) markedly reduced the emetic response to emetic agents acting centrally (loperamide) or peripherally (total-body radiation, intragastric copper sulphate) [2]. It was proposed that the blockade was due to a release and subsequent depletion of substance P or CGRP in the nucleus tractus solitarius in the brain stem. In the past few years, a number of animal studies (in ferret, dog, cat, house musk shrew) have been published demonstrating that selective nonpeptide antagonists for the neurokinin-1 (NK_1) receptor (one of the receptors at which substance P or a closely related substance acts) have the ability to block the retching and vomiting response to a wide variety of emetic stimuli, including cisplatin, radiation, apomorphine, intragastric copper sulphate, and motion [14, 15, 36, 38]. Thus they can block the responses to stimuli acting centrally and peripherally, which gives them a clear potential clinical advantage over the 5-HT_3 receptor antagonists. It is suggested that the antiemetic effect of the NK_1 receptor antagonists is due to antagonism of the action of substance P at a critical point in the emetic pathway, probably the NTS [38]. To date, there is no evidence that NK_1 receptor antagonists affect any other reflexes that involve the NTS. It is proposed that antagonists of the human NK1 receptor offer the best novel approach to complete blockade of retching and vomiting. However, it is not possible to comment on their efficacy against nausea, as this cannot be assessed directly in animals (it is a subjective sensation), and because of this the results of clinical studies are eagerly awaited, not only to see whether these agents offer a way forward but also to help better define the predictability (or otherwise) of the animal models of nausea and emesis.

Proposals for Clinical Studies that Would Facilitate Understanding of the Neuropharmacology of Emesis

Pharmacological Characterization of Antiemetic Failures

The question of whether failure is due to an inadequate (or inappropriate) drug or to the patient is, somewhat surprisingly, still unresolved. This question has two components. First, studies can only be undertaken in patients who have had optimal antiemetic treatment (i.e., a 5-HT_3 receptor antagonist and a steroid) for the acute phase of their first course of cytostatic therapy. The rationale for this is outlined above, and on scientific grounds it is indefensible to use suboptimal therapy on the first course of treatment and "wait for the patient to fail". If this comes about, such patients may have a problem (e.g., anticipatory emesis) not amenable to anything other than behavioral therapy. If a patient fails on a pharmacologically well-defined agent (e.g., a 5-HT_3 receptor antagonist), then by judicious use of other equally well-defined agents (e.g., domperidone, as opposed to prochlorperazine), progress will be made in teasing out the neuropharmacology of the pathways in different patient populations. If a non-systematic approach is used, we believe this is a retrogressive step, returning to the of polypharmacy era, with regimens involving multiple drugs, each with multiple actions. Our consensus is that this is not progress. However, we recognise that in man, for total control of emesis and perhaps even more of nausea, it may be be necessary to block a number of different brain stem receptor sites.

Dexamethasone: The Cenerentola of Antiemesis

It can be argued that the only disadvantage of dexamethasone is its low cost. Because of this, while it has demonstrable efficacy, there is little interest in understanding the mechanism of action, as there may be little to be gained (financially) by making a "better" dexamethasone. Pharmacologically, dexamethasone is a fascinating agent, because of its ability to enhance the antiemetic efficacy of diverse antiemetic agents (e.g., ondansetron [32]). While basic studies are revealing novel actions of dexamethasone (e.g., a possible neuroprotective action against cisplatin, [35]), virtually nothing is known about the mechanism of its antiemetic effects. This is perhaps best exemplified by the absence of a dose–response curve for dexamethasone. Such information is needed urgently, as it would presumably provide important insights into its mechanism. The efficacy of dexamethasone in delayed emesis is of particular interest, as it may indicate whether an inflammatory process is involved in the delayed phase of emesis.

What Is the True Spectrum of Antiemetic Action of the 5-HT$_3$ Receptor Antagonists?

The clinical efficacy of 5-HT$_3$ receptor antagonists against cytostatic anticancer therapy is not in doubt. A predominantly peripheral site of action (vagal afferents) with a central contribution for some compounds is consistent with this spectrum of action. However, it should also be noted that there are preliminary indications from over 20 studies (many uncontrolled) that a 5-HT$_3$ receptor antagonist (ondansetron) has some efficacy in ameliorating the nausea and vomiting caused by drug-induced gastric irritation, obstruction or distension, uremia, neurological trauma, and the carcinoid syndrome (e.g., [7, 17, 26, 34]). This antiemetic potential is worthy of much more detailed investigation in the cancer patient, with or without chemotherapy.

Patient Predictive Factors

In some ways, this aspect is the most amenable to study and may provide significant insights into the endogenous factors that determine individual emetic sensitivity. For example, ferrets challenged with apomorphine show different intensities of emetic response [11]. Humans also show differing sensitivity to emetic challenge. Thus women who show sensitivity to the nausea and emesis-inducing effects of the contraceptive pill show a clear trend to a greater and consistent incidence of nausea and vomiting during pregnancy and to travel sickness and migraine [39]. Pharyngeal stimulation can readily evoke the gag reflex in some people and not in others. Female sex hormones may alter the threshold of the emetic reflex [4, 8, 28]. Nausea and vomiting decrease with age [29], and, generally speaking, women appear to be more sensitive to nausea and/or emesis than men.

There have been no systematic attempts to compare gender differences in establishing a simple behavioral profile or emetogenic/nausea challenge that would be revealing of emetic sensitivity. Success here would be a major advance in better prediction of an effective use of costly medication.

References

1. Andrews PLR (1996) The mechanism of emesis induced by chemotherapy and radiotherapy, pp 3–24. In: Tonato M (ed) Anti-emetics in the supportive care of patients. (ESO monograph) Springer, Berlin Heidelberg New York
2. Andrews PLR, Bhandari PB (1993) Resinferatoxin, an ultrapotent capsaicin analogue, has anti-emetic properties in the ferret. Neuropharmacology 32 : 799–806
3. Andrews PLR, Davis CJ (1995) The physiology of emesis induced by anti-cancer therapy. In: Reynolds J, Andrews PLR, Davis CJ (eds) Serotonin and the scientific basis of anti-emetic therapy. Oxford Clinical Communications, Oxford, pp 25–49
4. Andrews PLR, Whitehead SA (1990) Pregnancy sickness. News Physiol Sci 5 : 5–10
5. Andrews PLR, Rapeport G, Sanger GJ (1988) Neuropharmacology of emesis induced by anti-cancer therapy. Trends Pharmacol Sci 9 : 334–341
6. Andrews PLR, Bhandari PB, Davis CJ (1992) Plasticity and modulation of the emetic reflex. In: Bianchi AL, Grelot L, Miller AD, King GI (eds) Mechanisms and control of emesis. John Libbey Eurotext, vol 223, INSERM, Paris, pp 275–284
7. Andrews PLR, Quan V, Ogg CS (1995) Ondansetron for symptomatic relief in terminal uraemia. Nephrol Dial Transplant 10 : 40
8. Beattie WS, Lindblad Z, Buckley ND, Forrest JB (1991) The incidence of postoperative nausea and vomiting in women undergoing laparoscopy is influenced by the day of the menstrual cycle. Can J Anaesth 38 : 298–302
9. Bruera E, Catz Z, Hooper R, Lentle B, MacDonald W (1987) Chronic nausea and anorexia in advanced cancer patients: a possible role for autonomic dysfunction. J Pain Symptom Manage 2 : 19–21
10. Costall B, Domeney AM, Naylor RJ, Tattersall FD (1986) 5-Hydroxytryptamine M-receptor antagonism to prevent cisplatin-induced emesis. Neuropharmacology 25 : 959–961
11. Costall B, Naylor RJ, Owera-Atepo J, Tattersall FD (1989) The responsiveness of the ferret to apomorphine-induced emesis. Br J Pharmacol 96 : 329P
12. Cubeddu LX, Alfieri AB, Hoffmen IS (1995) Clinical evidence for the involvement of serotonin in acute cytotoxic-induced emesis. In: Reynolds J, Andrews PLR, Davis CJ (eds) Serotonin and the scientific basis of anti-emetic therapie. Oxford Clinical Communications, Oxford pp 142–149
13. Cubeddu LX, O'Connor DT, Hoffmann I, Palmer RJ (1995) Plasma chromogranin A marks emesis and serotonin release associated with dacarbazine and nitrogen mustard but not with cyclophosphamide-based chemotherapies. Br J Cancer 72 : 1033–1038
14. Gardner CJ, Twissel DJ, Dale TJ, Gale JD, Jordan CC, Kilpatrick GJ, Bountra C, Ward P (1995) The broad spectrum anti-emetic activity of the novel non-peptide tachykinin NK-1 receptor antagonist GR 203040. Br J Pharmacol 116 : 158–163
15. Gonsalves S, Watson JW, Ashton C (1996) Broad spectrum antiemetic effect of CP-122 721, a tachykinin NK1 receptor antagonist, in ferrets. Eur J Pharmacol 305 : 181–185
16. Grelot L, Milano S, Le Stunff H (1995) Does 5HT play a role in the delayed phase of cisplatin-induced emesis? In: Reynolds J, Andrews PLR, Davis CJ (eds) Serotonin and

the scientific basis of anti-emetic therapy. Oxford Clinical Communications, Oxford, pp 181–191

17. Kleinerman KB, Deppe SA, Sargent AI (1993) Use of ondansetron for control of projectile vomiting in patients with neurosurgical trauma: two case reports. Ann Pharmacother 27 : 566–568

18. Lucot JB, Crampton GH (1989) 8-0H-DPAT suppresses vomiting in the cat elicited by motion cisplatin or xylazine. Pharmacol Biochem Behav 33 : 627–631

19. Matsuki N, Torii Y, Saito H (1993) Effects of iron and desferrioxamine on cisplatin-induced emesis: further evidence for the role of free radicals. Eur J Pharmacol [Environ Toxicol Pharmacol] 248 : 329–331

20. Miller AD; Jakus J, Nonaka S (1994) Plasticity of emesis to a 5HT-3 agonist: effect of visceral nerve cuts. Neuroreport 5 : 986–988

21. Miller AD, Rowley HA, Roberts PL, Kucharczyk J (1996) Human cortical activity during vestibular and drug-induced nausea detected using MSI. Ann NY Acad Sci 781 : 670–672

22. Miner WJ, Sanger GJ (1986) Inhibition of cisplatin induced vomiting by selective 5-hydroxytryptamine M-receptor antagonism. Br J Pharmacol 88 : 497–499

23. Minton AU, Swift N, Lawlor R, Mant C, Henry J (1995) Ipecacuanha-induced emesis – a human model for testing antiemetic drug activity. Clin Pharmacol Ther 54 : 53–57

24. Okada F, Saito H, Matsuki N (1995) Blockade of motion- and cisplatin-induced emesis by a 5-HT2 receptor agonist in Suncus murinus. Br J Pharmacol 114 : 931

25. Racke K, Schworer H, Kilbinger H (1995) The pharmacology of 5-HT release from enterochromaffin cells. In: Reynolds J, Andrews PLR, Davis CJ (eds) Serotonin and the scientific basis of anti-emetic therapy. Oxford Clinical Communications, Oxford, pp 84–89

26. Reed MD, Marx CM (1994) Ondansetron for treating nausea and vomiting in the poisoned patient. Ann Pharmacother 28 : 331–333

27. Reynolds DJM, Barber NA, Grahame-Smith DG, Leslie RA (1991) Cisplatin-evoked induction of c-fos protein in the brainstem of the ferret: the effect of cervical vagotomy and the anti-emetic 5HT-3 receptor antagonist granisetron (BRL43694). Brain Res 565 : 321–236

28. Roila F, Tonato M, Basurto C (1987) Antiemetic activity of high doses of metoclopramide combined with methylprednisolone versus metoclopramide alone in cisplatin treated cancer patients, a randomized double-blind trial of the Italian oncology group for clinical research. J Clin Oncol 5 : 141–149

29. Rub R, Andrews PLR, Whitehead SA (1992) Vomiting: incidence, causes, ageing and sex. In: Bianchi AL, Grelot L, Miller AD, King GI (eds) Mechanisms and control of emesis. (John Libbey Eurotext, vol 223) INSERM, Paris

30. Rudd JA, Naylor RJ (1993) The effect of 5-HT1A receptor ligands on copper sulphate-induced emesis in the ferret. Br J Pharmacol 100 : 99P

31. Rudd J, Naylor RJ (1994) Effects of 5HT-3 receptor antagonists on models of acute and delayed emesis induced by cisplatin in the ferret. Neuropharmacology 33 : 1607–1608

32. Rudd JA, Naylor RJ (1996) An interaction of ondansetron and dexamethasone antagonising cisplatin-induced acute and delayed emesis in the ferret. Br J Pharmacol 118 : 209–214

33. Rudd JA, Jordan CC, Naylor RJ (1996) The action of the NK1 tachykinin receptor antagonist CP99 994, in antagonising the acute and delayed emesis induced by cisplatin in the ferret. Br J Pharmacol 119 : 931–936

34. Schwörer H, MÅnke H, Stockmann F (1995) Treatment diarrhea in carcinoid syndrome with ondansetron, tropisetron and clonidine. Am J Gastroenterol 90 : 645–648
35. Scott RH, Woods AJ, Lacey MJ, Fernando D, Crawford JH, Andrews PLR (1995) An electrophysiological investigation into the effects of cisplatin and the protective effects of dexamethasone on cultured dorsal root ganglion neurones from neonatal rats. NS Arch Pharmacol 352 : 247–255
36. Tattersall FD, Rycroft W, Hill RG, Hargreaves RJ (1994) Enantioselective inhibition of apomorphine-induced emesis in the ferret by the neurokinin-1 receptor antagonist CP-99 994. Neuropharmacology 33 : 259–260
37. Tonini M (1995) 5HT4 receptor involvement in emesis. In: Reynolds J, Andrews PLR, Davis CJ (eds) Serotonin and the scientific basis of anti-emetic therapy. Oxford Clinical Communications, Oxford, pp 192–199
38. Watson JW, Gonsalves SF, Fossa AA, McLean S, Seeger T, Obach S, Andrews PLR (1995) The anti-emetic effects of CP-99 994 in the ferret and the dog: role of the NK1 receptor. Br J Pharmacol 115 : 84–94
39. Whitehead SA, Holden WA, Andrews PLR (1992) Pregnancy sickness. In: Bianchi AL, Grelot L, Miller AD, King GL (eds) Mechanisms and control of emesis. Libbey Eurotext, pp 297–306 (Colloque INSERM vol 223)